PAINFUL CHOICES

PAINFUL CHOICES

Research and Essays on Health Care

David Mechanic

Transaction Publishers
New Brunswick (U.S.A.) and Oxford (U.K.)

Copyright © 1989 by Transaction Publishers
New Brunswick, New Jersey 08903

Library of Congress Catalog Number: 88-24776
ISBN: 0-88738-258-4
Printed in the United States of America

Library of Congress Cataloging in Publication Data
Mechanic, David, 1936–
    Painful choices : research and essays on health care / David Mechanic.
        p.   cm.
    Includes bibliographies.
    ISBN 0-88738-258-4
    1. Medical care—United States.   2. Medical policy—United States.   3. Social medicine—United States.   I. Title.
    [DNLM: 1. Delivery of Health Care—United States.   2. Health Policy—United States.   3. Social Medicine—United States.   W 84 AA1 M48p]
RA445.M37   1989
362.1′0973—dc19
DNLM/DLC
for Library of Congress   88-24776
                                                                      CIP

For Gladys

Contents

Preface

The most important issue that concerns us in health care—how to provide accessible and effective care at affordable cost in an equitable way—has been on the agenda since early in this century and will occupy us for decades into the future. The current attention to changes in health care financing and regulation gives us the impression that the dilemmas we face are entirely new. The most central challenges, in contrast, are deep and persistent. While we may pose the problems in different ways at varying points in time, professional and organizational structures, American culture, and the dialectic between individual and collective responsibility are enduring themes.

This book brings together a selection of seventeen papers written during the past couple of decades, with a new introduction. The introduction, and the essays on challenges and choices, are all recent. But as I have reviewed the papers I have written over a longer period, I have been impressed more by the continuity of concerns and the enduring quality of the deeper issues than by the surface changes that occupy so much of contemporary commentary on the health scene. The papers on perspectives and approaches, and on research applications, in their essential qualities, are even more relevant today than when they were written. Their longevity, I believe, comes from the fact that they deal with fundamental questions and challenges and not simply with concerns of the moment.

In the earlier essays, especially, I am embarrassed by my dependence on male personal pronouns. The fact that these references seem so grating to me suggests improved sensitivity to such matters. Rather than modifying every such reference, I've left them as they originally were. It should be understood in every case that the references speak to humankind and not to gender.

In bringing these papers together, I am particularly grateful to Karen Orlando, who ably assisted me in the various tasks, such as proofreading, required to bring a manuscript to press.

Acknowledgments

The following articles and papers, which I have written previously, have been adapted for use in this book with permission from the original publishers:

Chapter 3 ("Sociological Critics versus Institutional Elites in the Politics of Research Application: Examples from Medical Care," in *Social Policy and Sociology*, ed. N. J. Demerath III, Otto Larsen, and Karl Schuessler [New York: Academic Press], 99–108); Chapter 4 ("The Concept of Illness Behavior: Culture, Situation and Personal Predisposition," *Psychological Medicine*, 16 [1986]: 1–7, with permission of Cambridge University Press); Chapter 5 ("Health and Behavior: Perspectives on Risk Prevention" reprinted from *Prevention in Health Psychology*, ed. James C. Rosen and Laura J. Solomon, by permission of University Press of New England, © 1985 by the Vermont Conference on the Primary Prevention of Psychopathology); Chapter 6 ("Social Structure and Personal Adaptation: Some Neglected Dimensions," pp. 32–44, from *Coping and Adaptation*, ed. George V. Coelho, David A. Hamburg, and John E. Adams. Copyright © 1974 by Basic Books, Inc. Reprinted by permission of Basic Books, Inc., Publishers); Chapter 7 ("Social Psychologic Factors Affecting the Presentation of Bodily Complaints," *New England Journal of Medicine* 286 [May 1972]: 1132–39); Chapter 8 ("Patient Behavior and the Organization of Medical Care," from *Ethics of Health Care*, ed. Lawrence R. Tancredi, by permission of the National Academy Press, 1974, pp. 67–85); Chapter 10 ("Development of Psychological Distress Among Young Adults," *Archives of General Psychiatry* 36 [October 1979]: 1233–39, © 1979, American Medical Association); Chapter 12 ("Distress Syndromes, Illness Behavior, Access to Care and Medical Utilization in a Defined Population," [with Paul D. Cleary and James Greenley] *Medical Care* 20 [April 1982]: 361–72, © 1982 Lippincott/Harper and Row); Chapter 13 ("Alternatives to

Mental Hospital Treatment: A Sociological Perspective," ed. Leonard T. Stein and Mary Ann Test [New York: Plenum Publishing Corporation, 1978], 309–20.); Chapter 14 ("Improving the Care of Patients with Chronic Mental Illness" [with Linda H. Aiken], *New England Journal of Medicine* 317 [December, 1987]: 1634–38); Chapter 15 ("Challenges in Health and Longterm Care Policy," *Health Affairs* 6 [Summer 1987]: 22–34); Chapter 17 ("Future Challenges in Health and Health Care," proceedings of the American Academy of Physician Assistants Symposium, *The Future of Health Care: Challenges and Choices*, 1985, pp. 1–3). Other chapters also appeared in the *Milbank Quarterly*, chapters 1 & 2 and in the *Journal of Health and Social Behavior*, chapters 9 and 11 (with Ronald Angel).

Introduction

Despite enormous expenditures in health care, now in excess of half a trillion dollars, all is not well in the medical arena. The availability of high-quality facilities, the latest technologies on the cutting edge, and an abundance of well-trained professionals should provide the conditions for a superb system of care, but the system itself is diminished by large gaps in entitlements and insurance; a lack of balance between curative efforts, rehabilitation, and prevention; and continuing failures to impose financial discipline on physicians, hospitals, and other service providers.

As government has become the major financial sponsor of health care through large insurance tax subsidies, the massive Medicare and Medicaid programs, and numerous other categorical entitlements, the burden of growing costs increasingly falls on the public. With a large federal deficit, and financial pressures on state and local government as well, vigorous regulatory efforts are now being made to limit costs. These intrusive efforts reflect the unwieldly organization of health services and are burdensome and costly to administer. Under the guise of maintaining a private-sector industry, the United States has evolved the most elaborate, and increasingly cumbersome, framework for the financing and regulation of health services in the world. As each new problem gains visibility, from cost to quality of outcome, the typical wisdom is to introduce more and more regulatory requirements.

Though the size of the administrative infrastructure in the United States is remarkable, it is taken for granted by most of the population. One report in the *New England Journal of Medicine* estimated that $77.7 billion dollars was spent in 1983 on health care administration, 22 percent of all expenditures for health care in that year.[1] One can easily quarrel with the estimate, but not with the fact that administration consumes a significant component of total expenditures. The administrative costs of maintaining the type of

1

decentralized, service-driven payment that characterizes health insurance in America are awesome, and while the arrangement creates some employment, it contributes relatively little to health. Between 1970 and 1982, total health care personnel increased by 57 percent, but administrative personnel grew by 171 percent.[2] The mountains of paper that characterize the billing and accountability procedures we follow might be acceptable if they were in the cause of effective allocation of resources; unfortunately, they mirror the imbalances and absurdities of the health care arena itself. The patterns of payment and reimbursement that these administrative procedures support encourage an emphasis on curative efforts, no matter how remote, a bias toward inpatient care in hospitals and other institutions, and incentives to overuse sophisticated procedures and technology. In contrast, reimbursement incentives devalue necessary sociomedical care and rehabilitation, prevention, cognitive services and educational efforts, and a perspective that gives attention to enhancing the quality of life and function through the health services system.

Studies of the increasing use of heart-rate monitoring exemplifies the difficulty.[3] This technology, first introduced commercially in 1969, was quickly and widely adopted. Within two years, it was universally accepted in large teaching programs and was used routinely in most pregnancies, replacing the traditional method of auscultation. It also spread widely in general hospitals and was soon used in about half of all births. Initial uncontrolled studies suggested that the procedure had some value, but eight subsequent randomized controlled trials found no support for this claim. Monitoring may be associated with a slightly smaller probability of neonatal seizures, but it is unlikely overall to have any advantage. Electronic monitoring capability is seemingly impressive, but it is costly and provides little beyond traditional care in most instances. Moreover, because it occasionally results in exaggerated assessments of fetal distress, its consequence may be increased numbers of Cesarean sections and forceps deliveries. In addition, physicians and nurses are no longer taught traditional auscultation, making them totally dependent on electronic monitoring. Despite strong evidence that would discourage widespread use, the technologic imperative has persisted. In contrast, repeated studies emphasize the crucial importance of appropriate prenatal care in preventing infant death and morbidity—a simple, noninvasive, and inexpensive technology, easily applied.[4] But with all of our technological and organizational capacities, we seem unable or unwilling to bring these services to those at higher risk.

The above observations seem to apply broadly to the use of sophisticated electronics in medical care as opposed to the use of simpler, traditional techniques. Another widely diffused technology, intensive coronary care providing continuous electrocardiographic monitoring, is almost universally used despite several randomized controlled trials that showed no advantage, and one that actually indicated worse outcomes for some patient subgroups, when compared to home care.[5] These studies have not changed the basic pattern of technologic dependence, but they may have contributed to the fact that patients now spend less time in coronary care units. Electrocardiographic monitoring detects more arrhythmias, but these occur early after myocardial infarction, making long periods of intensive monitoring unnecessary for patients without major complications, and those without elevated total serum creatine phosphokinase or electrocardiographic evidence of early transmural infarction.[6]

Outside observers of our health care system are often astonished that we can spend so much and yet have such extraordinary gaps in access and quality of care. How does a system with such generous financing leave 37 million people uninsured? Having returned the mentally ill to communities, why do we then tolerate the extraordinary neglect that characterizes their care? How can a nation that makes war on drug abuse and the spread of AIDS fail to provide essential treatment to large numbers of addicts at risk of AIDS who seek assistance in breaking their habits? Why do we make so many services needed by the homebound elderly to enhance their independence and quality of life contingent upon admission to institutions? Why are our efforts to appropriately immunize our children, to correct child health problems before they become chronic, and to prevent subsequent morbidity and disability so fragmented?

The failure is not in our understanding, our awareness of the problems and challenges, or even our sympathies. The barrier most typically is how we make decisions about money, and the unwillingness of policymakers to augment already large commitments to the health care sector. Looking at overall expenditures, it seems incredible that we cannot make significant progress in solving these problems, but the issues are typically not conceptualized in these terms. There are already strong interests to defend existing priorities and reimbursement patterns, and thus it becomes exceedingly difficult to have a meaningful public discussion of trade-offs. Whenever serious efforts are made to address allocation issues, the interests involved have an extraordinary capacity to "cry wolf" and alarm the public. Hospitals, for example, were making increased profits during the period they were vociferously claiming that Diagnostic Related Groups (DRGs) were destroying their sector. The result is that the politics of meeting needs is defined commonly in terms of augmenting existing expenditures without altering the status quo or existing incentives. The cost implications, of course, frighten prudent policymakers.

It is increasingly evident that we cannot solve the health care problems we face without significantly restructuring how we finance and organize medical services. From a governmental perspective, the highest priority is to put a lid on growing expenditures and, if possible, to address some of the glaring inequities as well. The inescapable conclusion is that there is a need for a controllable prospective budget. The public sector clearly has been moving in this direction through the establishment of DRGs for hospital reimbursement under Medicare, the promotion of Health Maintenance Organizations (HMOs), and demonstrations under Medicare and Medicaid using the waiver authority of the Health Care Financing Administration. In each case, the efforts are too modest in intent, and not at the scale necessary to achieve needed transformations.

The implementation of DRGs is a case in point. Seeking to correct the consequences of open-ended budgeting characteristic of cost reimbursement, the Medicare program now pays hospitals on the basis of 468 DRGs that provide a predetermined payment for patients admitted with a particular illness pattern. Within specified parameters, the payment remains the same regardless of the length of stay or the intensity of care. The intent is to eliminate the incentive for excessive and often unnecessary care by allowing hospitals to retain savings from DRG reimbursement but be at risk for care beyond the predetermined payment. Pricing of the various DRGs becomes the lever that gives government the potential to contain costs, provided it has the capacity to resist political pressures from powerful hospital and medical technology industries for more advantageous pricing.

A major limitation of DRGs is their restriction to inpatient care, in contrast to the total care during an illness episode. This encourages "gaming" among providers. In response to DRGs, the site of service for various diagnostic and surgical procedures has shifted to outpatient settings where costs are not controlled in comparable ways. Further, some aspects of care typical of inpatient care previously provided on an inpatient basis have been shifted to the prehospital and posthospital stages, which are separately reimbursed. This is not necessarily inconsistent with regulatory intent, particularly if aggregate costs decrease; but many of the costs have simply been shifted from hospitals to other sectors. It has been alleged that patients are discharged "quicker and sicker," although the evidence to sustain the claim on a broad basis has been lacking. If hospitals discharge patients when they should remain in the hospital, one would expect more frequent readmissions, which would also increase hospital payment, a pattern that must then be monitored. Moreover, a fixed reimbursement per admission provides incentives for marginal admissions if they are not controlled through utilization review or in other ways. Government studies suggest that approximately 10 percent of Medicare admissions fit this picture. Most serious from a quality-of-care perspective is the almost exclusive focus on the inpatient part of an illness episode, with resultant neglect of what happens before and after. Thus far, there is no persuasive evidence that DRGs have had any substantial effect on aggregate costs.

This halfway approach to prospective budgeting has had other costs as well. Policymakers are not unsophisticated, and they anticipated the change of incentives and much of the "gaming" that resulted. The response, as we might have anticipated, has been the development of new regulations that close the loopholes, more intensive monitoring of the need for hospitalization by professional review organizations, and the like. In each case, the regulatory mechanisms appear suitable, but in their totality they are incredibly costly.

The concomitant strategy, the encouragement of HMOs, has the fundamental advantage that financing is tied to defined populations and covers the range of usual inpatient and outpatient services. Capitating enrollees— that is, paying a predetermined fixed amount for their total care—provides an opportunity to trade outpatient for inpatient care, marginally useful technical procedures for preventive and educational activities, and the like. There is impressive evidence that HMOs use less hospital care, significantly reducing total costs. Thus, it becomes possible to capitate enrollees for their total medical care for less cost than would be incurred through the conventional pattern of medical services. In the case of public programs such as Medicaid and Medicare, eligible recipients can be enrolled at less than the average cost for public recipients in their geographic area. When it uses such insurance plans instead of cost reimbursements, the government is only at risk for the premium cost and, thus, can project costs in advance.

HMOs, originally, were modeled on the large nonprofit prepaid group practices such as Kaiser-Permanente and Group Health Insurance, organizations that had established leadership, philosophies, and well-established operating procedures. As the competitive initiative gained momentum in the 1980s, and as HMO enrollment grew, many organizations, both profit and nonprofit, lacking comparable leadership and care philosophies proliferated. Moreover, because patients resisted closed-panel HMOs that restricted utilization to a limited number of physicians, much of the later growth was in newly established Independent Practice Associations that were prepaid but allowed a much broader scope of physician choice. But much of what we know about the performance of HMOs is based on the older, more established, prepaid group practices rather than on these newer entities. Moreover, as the HMO sector grew, more abuses became evident.

From a governmental perspective, the fact that recipients in such programs as Medicare have a choice of usual care versus HMOs results in some special difficulties. In the early history of HMOs, there was considerable speculation that these organizations would attract persons in need of more care because the coverage was comprehensive and minimized the need for additional out-of-pocket expenditures. Overall, there was no consistent or persuasive evidence of such "risk vulnerability," and experience suggested that HMOs could function more economically than the dominant fee-for-service sector with comparable patients.[7] Moreover, the Rand Health Insurance Experiment demonstrated that these cost advantages persisted even when patients were randomized among alternative insurance plans, eliminating selection effects.[8] As researchers began studying the experience of elders in HMOs, some found that those who joined these types of organizations had lower levels of hospital utilization in the period prior to joining than nonenrollees.[9] This suggested that HMOs were attracting older persons of lower risk and those who should cost less to serve than the typical nonenrollee.

The research on this issue is still fragmentary, and the evidence is less than fully persuasive. But it seems plausible that the sick elderly, who may have developed intensive relationships with specific physicians on whom they have become dependent, might be particularly reluctant to leave these relationships for an alternative care arrangement. Risk selection, as this issue is called, is of importance because if HMOs attract persons of lesser risks, they are likely to be overpaid for the enrollees they serve. More crucial, if such selection occurs, the aggregate costs of the Medicare program could be larger than before. One might suspect that the marketing strategy of HMOs—particularly the more profit-oriented ones—would be directed to the lower-risk enrollee. On the other side of the ledger is the fact that some HMOs are leaving the Medicare business, maintaining that reimbursement is too low to cover the required care. One solution to these selection issues, now being worked on, is to relate the premium the government will pay to an estimate of need for care. The techniques, and validity of such estimates remain uncertain, however, and it may be costly to adequately assess risk on an individual basis. If membership in HMOs was universally mandated, the selection issue would disappear, but such restriction of choice in the Medicare program would be viewed by many as unacceptable.

The Medicaid program, developing out of a welfare perspective, has more aggressively imposed restrictions on choice. Some states, for example, mandate HMO enrollment or have developed systems of preferred providers who agree to render needed services to Medicaid recipients at an agreed-upon price. Other factors comparable, restriction of choice has disadvantages in that satisfaction is likely to be higher when people choose their source of care, and this encourages a stronger professional-patient relationship. In contrast, if economies are achieved by restrictions in choice in public programs, and these economies are translated into more comprehensive benefits or increased coverage of the poor population, then the trade-off might be an advantageous one. Medicaid has not kept pace with the level of poverty in the population, and less than half of those meeting federal poverty criteria are eligible for this program. It is the population that is too poor to purchase private insurance but not eligible for public subsidy that is critical for social policy.

From the government's point of view, HMOs have the additional advantage of a predetermined cap on the payment for each enrollee, with no need for detailed regulation at a microlevel. Government thus achieves its objective of budgetary planning and staying within a predictable budget for HMO enrollees without the need to monitor the appropriateness of hospital admissions, procedures, and the like. When there are allegations of financial irregularities or that essential services are being withheld, it is necessary to intrude into the plans involved, but the HMO framework, in general, provides a context requiring much less intrusion than traditional care.

Despite the rapid growth of HMOs in the 1980s, this form of practice has been disappointing to many of its longtime advocates. The early history of HMOs was often linked to a patient care philosophy that has eroded as new profit-oriented entrepreneurs have moved into this arena. Moreover, while the advantage of HMOs in reducing hospital admissions and surgical interventions persist, there is little evidence that the basic orientations and patterns of patient care are different from those found in other care contexts. HMOs have traditionally been attractive to young families that need routine care but have little serious illness. As HMO members age, however, the prevalence of serious illness and the management of appropriate care for this older HMO population are not so easily dealt with. Many people who anticipate the need for complicated services are skeptical that HMOs will truly meet their needs, and there is resistance to HMO enrollment among them. As HMOs have competed for enrollees in an increasingly competitive marketplace, they have reduced premiums by cutting back on benefits for particular services, such as psychiatric illness. The consequence is that HMOs are not likely to offer such patients the services and protections they need. Some argue that this is the case for many other chronic diseases as well.[10] The fact is that many HMOs do not particularly want these enrollees because they have complicated needs and are costly to manage appropriately. With financial pressures on the entire health arena, and a trend toward less hospital care, the magnitude of the HMOs' economic advantage as a result of reduced hospitalization may erode over time.

As profit has become a more important element in HMOs, there are increased pressures on physicians to ration care rigorously. In earlier HMOs, savings primarily came by reducing hospital care and surgical interventions, but patterns of outpatient practice styles were comparable to the fee-for-service sector. But, increasingly, HMO administrators are making new efforts to constrain physician behavior. A most serious change is to put the individual physicians' remuneration at risk when they exceed particular cost targets. In earlier efforts to develop incentives for efficiency and resource conservation, some group practices established a general fund that would be shared by physicians if costs were successfully constrained, but the incentive for any single physician was not so large as to have much chance of influencing clinical decisions and loyalty to patients. Some of the new incentives being developed are far more forceful and put the interests of the physician and the patient at odds. Defining appropriate and inappropriate incentives is a crucial issue as new delivery systems evolve.

As noted, one advantage of HMOs has been their ability to consider trade-offs among different components of medical care. But as we must care for larger numbers of frail elderly and others with serious chronic disease, we need to transcend a narrow definition of medical care and also consider trade-offs with other services essential to maintaining function, independent living, and quality of life. Long-term care is one of the largest problem areas our health care system faces, and new ways must be developed to expand services to encompass these needs. In doing so, we must deal with the issue of financing such care for the population at risk as well as with the issue of organization of appropriate delivery systems. The Social Health Maintenance Organization (SHMO) begins to address the latter issue.

The SHMO, currently being evaluated in a demonstration project financed by the Health Care Financing Administration at four sites, seeks to achieve a better balance between traditional medical care services, home care, and needed social services.[11] The SHMO offers a variety of medical and social services within a managed care system expanding benefits to include homemakers, home health and chore services, meals, counseling, and transportation. Depending on the plan, the range of services may be very broad, limited only by financing and the organization's ability to provide or coordinate services through its own delivery system or through contracting. Each of the four demonstration SHMOs presently being studied has a different sponsor and varying expanded-care benefits, premium structures, and selection criteria for providing these expanded benefits. As several of the chapters in this volume show, the challenge of chronic disease and long-term care requires an expanded framework of care that brings together the elements necessary to sustain function and community adaptation.

Financing, of course, is a key element in determining what we can accomplish. The fact that the United States is the only major Western nation that lacks a health insurance system covering its entire population is widely noted. While we have fragments of such a system in place through Medicare and Medicaid, and tax incentives for employers to subsidize insurance to workers, we have enormous unfilled gaps. In the 1970s, the nation came close to enacting a national health insurance plan; only the inability to gain support from organized labor, which advocated a more radical plan, doomed an emerging consensus. As fiscal problems have mounted in recent years, the country has turned away from this issue. Discussion of national health insurance is likely to return to the national agenda in coming years because existing deficiencies in coverage are of increasing concern to the Congress, to the business establishment, and to the hospital industry, as well as to the usual advocacy groups. The problem of inadequate insurance creates enormous pressures on many hospitals that provide a great deal of uncompensated care, and growing awareness of lack of equity in access has led to concern among increasing numbers of the American public.

In recent decades, we learned the lesson that simply expanding insurance coverage without a framework of controls leads to extraordinary cost increases. Although many Americans abhor the notion of rationing, which evokes in their minds the queues and allocations associated with war, there is growing realization that a more obvious rationing framework will be required if we are ever to ensure an equitable system of care. I first raised this issue and suggested a theory of rationing in an article published in the *Milbank Memorial Quarterly* more than a decade ago (see chapter 1). Since then, a fairly large literature has evolved, reflecting policy analysts' growing awareness of its inevitability.[12]

One factor making conscious rationing inevitable is the extraordinary growth of biomedical science and sophisticated technology that seems to open never-ending possibilities for extending function and life. The transplantation of kidneys and bone marrow have become almost routine, and the transplantation of livers, hearts, and lungs are not too far behind. Impressive progress is being made in the transplantation of tissue in the brain in animal models, and already such approaches have been used in surgical intervention for Parkinson's disease. The growing pressures on the Medicare program are in part a product of new and impressive technologies such as computerized tomography (CT) and nuclear magnetic resonance (NMR) imaging devices, coronary angioplasty and open heart surgery, implantation of intraocular lenses, total hip replacement, and, most recently, shock-wave lithotripsy. Many of these technologies involve enormous capital investments, but they also frequently substitute for more invasive interventions and contribute importantly to health when used appropriately.

We have not been particularly successful in regionalizing these very sophisticated and expensive technologies, and many hospitals acquire them for reasons of prestige, competitiveness with other hospitals, or potential for profit. The need then is to amortize these expensive investments, and the technology comes to be used in many instances when it is not essential or even appropriate, in part to generate income. There is much agreement among experts that restricting many of these new technologies to centers with high volume is efficient, and it may be conducive to better care as well. Centers with high volume in the use of complex specialized techniques develop the experience and have the capacity to maintain the range of expertise essential to high-quality care.

The problem remains how best to take advantage of the benefits of new technologies without promiscuous diffusion, inappropriate use, and budgetary excesses. The issue, then, turns explicitly to the criteria for allocation and the types of technologies for which government programs and health insurance plans should pay. One technique used by Medicare for some highly expensive procedures is to restrict payment to hospitals that maintain a sufficient volume of these procedures. A danger in this approach is that it creates strong incentives to do these procedures in uncertain cases. Much of the effectiveness of medical care and the use of technology is uncertain, and the data on utilization in uncertain instances show enormous variations from one geographic area to another.[13] Unfortunately, we have no clear way of defining what level of utilization is most appropriate, and while cost-conscious policymakers might want to use the lower levels characteristic of some geographic areas as the criterion, it is unlikely that this is the appropriate standard.

There is much evidence of unnecessary and inappropriate care, but the issue of concern is much larger. In many instances, the value of technology and specific medical and surgical procedures is highly uncertain and the data to evaluate the efficacy and cost-effectiveness of varying types of care are not available.[14] It is this large region of uncertainty, and the lack of clear norms, that gives clinical discretion such influence and justifies in the minds of many physicians the extraordinary variations that are routinely reported. There is growing consciousness of these problems in the medical arena, but physicians have not been strong advocates of the types of scientific studies that can help resolve some of these issues. Instead, they fall back on their clinical experience and often give this more credence than results from well-designed investigations.

Some have argued that certain very costly technologies benefiting few persons, such as heart transplants, should not be made available, but there is a strong political impetus to cover such procedures in insurance programs as the technology is perfected and outcomes improve. The American public has great faith in technology and will not easily accept the view that efficacious technologies should be withheld. The rationing that is most likely to be implemented on a widespread basis involves decisions among technologies that have comparable functions but vary widely in cost. In recent years, for example, progress has been made in the development of thrombolytic agents, drugs that dissolve blood clots, administered to patients after heart attacks. The drug of choice has been streptokinase, but Genentech, using genetic engineering techniques, has developed a new thrombolytic agent, tissue plasminogen activator (TPA), which some physicians would prefer because they believe it involves fewer side effects, although there is no firm evidence that the new drug is superior to the less-costly one. Since the potential Medicare population receiving these drugs is large, the relative costs of these alternative drugs become pertinent. TPA costs far more than comparable drugs—at present more than ten times as much—and the Medicare program has decided not to pay for it. While doctors complain of rationing by price and control over clinical decisions, the Health Care Financing Administration's decision seems fully defensible until such time as TPA is proved to be clearly advantageous in reducing mortality and morbidity or in preventing serious adverse effects. Moreover, even if there was a small advantage, the issue remains as to whether limited government resources should be invested in such increased expenditures.

A related issue concerns the appropriate indications for using a technology paid for by public programs. The implantation of permanent cardiac pacemakers is a relatively common procedure among the elderly covered by Medicare. Approximately 120,000 pacemakers are implanted annually in the United States, at an average cost of $12,000. It has been alleged for some time that a large proportion of implants under the Medicare program were unnecessary. In one recent study of the implantation of new pacemakers in 30 Philadelphia hospitals, the investigators examined patients' charts to assess whether the indications for implants were appropriate and adequately documented.[15] They found that one-fifth of the implants were not indicated on the basis of the information contained on the record, and another 36 percent were ambiguous. Inappropriate use of pacemakers was evident in all types of hospitals. It is not unreasonable for Medicare to set explicit standards for appropriate use of such procedures as a criterion for payment.

An alternative approach to rationing focuses less on the efficacy of particular procedures and technologies and more on the attributes of patients who might potentially receive them. These issues first came clearly into focus with the development of renal hemodialysis, which makes it possible for persons with end-stage renal disease to survive and continue functioning. Initially, the facilities were very limited relative to the potential recipient population, and efforts were made to allocate treatment on the basis of not only medical need and possible benefit but also on the alleged social and moral "worth" of potential recipients. The extraordinary conflict implicit in such decisions, and the potential for political pressures and interventions, quickly made clear the mischief inherent in such judgmental activities. In one instance, for example, the fact of church attendance favored one possible treatment recipient over another. In another case, the intervention of a U.S. senator who had some budgetary authority over the public facility resulted in a subterfuge to allow a preferred patient to jump the queue. The rapid growth and diffusion of hemodialysis facilities and the coverage of care for patients with end-stage renal disease under Medicare eliminated the pressures for rationing. As a matter of public policy, it remains unclear to what extent coverage of care for one disease but not others, where there may be comparable benefits, is wise. The problem, of course, is the political potency of public pleas for lifesaving technologies, which we see increasingly in the area of heart and liver transplants.

Among the personal qualities viewed as relevant to rationing, age is the one most commonly advocated as a basis for withholding care. Some other Western countries with more limited resources than the United States have been less willing to make expensive technologies such as hemodialysis available to all who might benefit.[16] In the English National Health Service, where such facilities have been limited, there is an understanding among doctors that persons over age fifty-five will not be dialyzed. There is no explicit rule, but the system functions so as to allow older patients with chronic renal failure to die. In the English view, the same scarce economic resources could be used with greater benefit for other health priorities.

There is not much chance that the type of rationing characteristic of the National Health Service would be acceptable to the American public. As new possibilities abound for extending life, however, there are increasing suggestions that age should be the basis for triage. It is not difficult to understand the thinking behind such advocacy, in that longevity is typically associated with more chronic illness, increasing disability, and high medical expenditures. Daniel Callahan, for example, has argued for the need to place limits "on the length of individual lives that a society can sensibly be expected to maintain at public cost."[17] He argues that we should desist from goals in which the elderly are primarily the beneficiaries, the costs are high, and gains for the entire population are marginally slight. He believes that we should view death as a condition of life to be accepted, "if not for our own sake, then at least for the sake of others."[18] It is arguable whether such rationing would save all that much money, but the idea has even more fundamental defects.

Age is perhaps an easier criterion to apply than others, but it shares the crudity of all such global distinctions that neglect individual differences and the variations in function and vitality, and goals and aspirations, among persons of comparable age. Age is connected with chronicity on a probabilistic basis, but using probabilistic statements to make individual decisions confuses background and information with moral decisions. It is well known, for example, that blacks commit many more crimes than whites in the United States, but could one reasonably argue that blacks have less right to be treated fairly by police and given due process than others? Age as a criterion, like any other ascriptive characteristic, is inherently discriminatory. However, efforts to develop allocation criteria that take into account medical likelihood of success, potential benefits and risks, and other such indicators are acceptable. And, indeed, such criteria may favor the young over the elderly in many instances. But such decisions are made on the basis of assessing the value of an intervention in relation to individual situations and facts and not simply on the basis of a categorical judgment. Our society, thus far, has not been forced to truly confront such issues in a major way, but more serious pressures along these lines are inevitable. There will be no way to avoid these painful choices.

In chapter 1, I present a portrait of the dynamics of medical technology and care organization and introduce some general theoretical approaches to the rationing issues. In the next two chapters, I address the role of social research in health care and health services, issues that are often troubling both to those who do such work and to those who fund it. Unlike work on specific diseases with which legislators can identify because of their own experiences with illness among family and friends, few can easily identify with research on health services itself. This results in instability in funding and an underlying insecurity about the future among researchers. The consequences, in turn, affect recruitment of talented persons and their commitment to the field. A related concern is the difficulty health services researchers have in influencing important health policy discussions, especially when the issue involves many strong interest groups and active political dialogue. Here I argue for a long-range perspective, one that is modest in its expectations that politicians will immediately use the findings of research but confident that good research affects how policymakers define issues over time and adopt health care strategies.

The next section of the book includes a selection of five chapters that reflect my way of viewing issues of health, help-seeking and the physician's response, and personal adaptation. In considering such issues as risk behavior and prevention, self-appraisal, utilization of medical care, and the physician's response to complex psychosocial factors, I illustrate how culture and social structure influence medical events, and how any fruitful understanding of individual and public health issues must take account of the social dimensions. Medical care is a behavioral system and cannot be understood outside a framework of expectations, norms, and cultural variabilities.

I then turn to research issues, presenting selected research studies that illustrate how the broader perspectives I gave are translated into research strategies and designs. The three research examples I supply reflect efforts to study the developmental determinants of distress syndromes in young adults; to understand why persons with comparable objective physical dysfunction relevant to back pain react differently in their appraisal and response patterns; and to examine how one might explain the high concordance in utilization of medical and psychiatric care. It should be evident how these studies arise from and inform the perspectives developed in the earlier section.

The chapters in the final section address some of the most critical issues in the future of health services. The first two deal with the extraordinary neglect of the most seriously mentally ill in our society, the difficulty of developing viable and effective alternatives to long-term hospitalization, and potential strategies for the future. The following chapter also deals with long-term care, but in relation to the growing elderly population. Long-term care of the elderly shares many of the financial and structural problems associated with care of chronic mental illness, but these problems involve much larger populations, and enormous expenditures. Thus, they are the focus of much greater public attention. I conclude the volume with a brief summary of future health challenges and a general philosophy of how we might best address them.

Notes

1. David Himmelstein and Steffie Woolhandler, "Cost Without Benefit: Administrative Waste in U.S. Health Care," *New England Journal of Medicine* 314 (1986): 441–46.
2. Ibid.
3. K. K. Shy, E. B. Larson, and D. A. Luthy, "Evaluating a New Technology:

The Effectiveness of Electronic Fetal Heart Rate Monitoring," *Annual Review of Public Health* 8 (1987): 165–90.

4. Institute of Medicine, *The Prevention of Low Birthweight* (Washington, D.C.: National Academy Press, 1985); Diane Dutton, "Social Class, Health, and Illness," in *Applications of Social Science to Clinical Medicine and Social Policy,* ed. L. H. Aiken and D. Mechanic (New Brunswick, N.J.: Rutgers University Press, 1986), 31–62.

5. Shy, Larson, and Luthy, "Evaluating a New Technology"; H. Waitzkin, "A Marxist Interpretation of the Growth and Development of Coronary Care Technology," *American Journal of Public Health* 69 (1979): 1260–68.

6. A. G. Mulley et al., "The Course of Patients With Suspected Myocardial Infarction: The Identification of Low-Risk Patients for Early Transfer From Intensive Care," *New England Journal of Medicine* 302 (1980): 943–48.

7. Harold S. Luft, *Health Maintenance Organizations: Dimensions of Performance* (New Brunswick, N.J.: Transaction Books, 1987).

8. W. Manning et al., "A Controlled Trial of the Effect of a Prepaid Group Practice on Use of Services," *New England Journal of Medicine* 310 (1984): 1505–10.

9. P. Eggers and R. Prihoda, "Pre-enrollment Reimbursement Patterns of Medicare Beneficiaries Enrolled in 'at risk' HMOs," *Health Care Financing Review* 4 (1982): 55–73.

10. Mark Schlesinger, "On the Limits of Expanding Health Care Reform: Chronic Care in Prepaid Settings," *The Milbank Quarterly* 64 (1986): 189–215.

11. Walter Leutz et al., "Targeting Expanded Care to the Aged: Early SHMO Experience," *The Gerontologist* 28 (1988): 4–17.

12. David Mechanic, *Future Issues in Health Care: Social Policy and the Rationing of Medical Services* (New York: The Free Press, 1979), and *From Advocacy to Allocation: The Evolving American Health Care System* (New York: The Free Press, 1986); J. H. Aaron and W. B. Schwartz, *The Painful Prescription: Rationing Health Care* (Washington, D.C.: Brookings Institute, 1984); Daniel Callahan, "Adequate Health Care and an Aging Society: Are They Morally Compatible?", *Daedalus* 115 (1986): 247–67; Robert Blank, *Rationing Medicine* (New York: Columbia University Press, 1988); Larry Churchill, *Rationing Health Care in America* (Notre Dame: University of Notre Dame Press, 1987).

13. J. Wennberg and S. Gittelsohn, "Small Area Variations in Health Care Delivery," *Science* 182 (1973): 1102–08; J. Wennberg, "Dealing with Medical Practice Variations: A Proposal for Action," *Health Affairs* 3 (1984): 6–32.

14. David Eddy and John Billings, "The Quality of Medical Evidence: Implications for Quality of Care," *Health Affairs* 7 (1988): 19–32.

15. A. M. Greenspan et al., "Incidence of Unwarranted Implantation of Permanent Cardiac Pacemakers in a Large Medical Population," *New England Journal of Medicine* 318 (1988): 158–163.

16. Aaron and Schwartz, *The Painful Prescription.*

17. Callahan, "Adequate Health Care," 266.

18. Ibid., 262.

19. For those interested in these problems in much greater depth, I suggest as supplemental reading my *Mental Health and Social Policy,* 3rd ed. (Englewood Cliffs, N.J.: Prentice Hall, 1989).

Part I
THE CHANGING HEALTH ARENA AND SOCIAL RESEARCH

1

The Growth of Medical Technology and Bureaucracy: Implications for Medical Care

Despite significant differences in ideology, values, and social organization, most Western developed countries—and probably most countries in the world—face common problems of financing, organizing, and providing health care services. As populations increasingly demand medical care, there is growing concern among the governments of most nations to provide a minimal level of service to all and to decrease obvious inequalities in care. To use available technology and knowledge efficiently and effectively, certain organizational options are most desirable. Thus, there is a general tendency throughout the world to link existing services to defined population groups, to develop new and more economic ways to provide primary services to the population without too great an emphasis on technological efforts, to integrate services increasingly fragmented by specialization or a more elaborate division of labor, and to seek ways to improve the output of the delivery system with fixed inputs. Although all of these concerns to some extent characterize national planning in underdeveloped countries, they particularly describe tendencies among developed countries as they attempt to control the enormous costs of available technologies. Throughout the world there is increasing movement away from medicine as a solitary entrepreneurial activity and more emphasis on the effective development of health delivery systems.

Having discussed these trends elsewhere in detail (Mechanic, 1974, 1976), what I will do here is examine how changing technology and organization affect not only the provision of medical care, but also the underlying assumptions of practitioners and patients. My thesis is that medical care constitutes a complex psychological system of assumptions and meanings that is significantly affected by the bureaucratization of medical tasks and the growing specification of the technical aspects. Public policies everywhere in the world increasingly play a role in the financing and organization of care, but when such public policies violate the psychological assumptions and social expectations of health practitioners and patients, they may have consequences very different from those intended.

Modes of Rationing Health Services

Medicine has in recent decades undergone an enormous development in specialized knowledge and in technology. While these advances have brought considerable progress in treating some diseases, most of the major diseases affecting mortality and morbidity—from heart disease and the cancers to the psychoses and substance abuse—are only poorly understood, and existing efforts, while they ameliorate suffering and sometimes extend life, are not able to cure or prevent the incidence of most of these conditions. The technologies that do exist are often extraordinarily expensive, require intensive professional manpower, and must be applied repeatedly to a patient during the long course of a chronic condition. Take an example where success has been quite impressive, such as in hemodialysis and transplantation in end-stage kidney disease: intensive and expensive efforts must be made over a long period to sustain life and functioning, which on a per capita basis consume a very high level of expenditure (Fox and Swazey, 1974). As these halfway technologies have developed—intensive care units, radiation therapy for cancers, coronary bypass surgery—the aggregate costs of medical care have continued to move upward, with medical services consuming a larger proportion of national income. In the United States, for example, where in 1940 the cost of health care was $4 billion and 4 percent of the gross national product, 1988 costs were about a half trillion dollars and 11 percent of the gross national product. While the proportional increase is not as large in nations having a centralized prospective budgeting process, as in England, the trend, nevertheless, is the same and a source of concern among all thoughtful people.

Since the prevalence of illness and "dis-ease" is extremely high in community populations, as has been repeatedly demonstrated by morbidity surveys (White et al., 1961), there is almost unlimited possibility for the continued escalation of medical demand and increased medical expenditures. As people have learned to have higher and more unrealistic expectations of medicine, demands for care for a wide variety of conditions, both major and minor, have accelerated. No nation that follows a sane public policy would facilitate the fulfillment of all perceptions of need that a demanding public might be willing to make. As in every other area of life, resources must be rationed. The uncontrolled escalation of costs in developed countries results in part because techniques of rationing are in a process of transition, and most countries have yet to reach a reasonable end point in this transitional process. The process is one of movement from *rationing by fee* through a stage of *implicit rationing* through resource allocation to a final stage of *explicit rationing*. In this process the role of physician shifts from entrepreneur to bureaucratic official, and medical practice from a market-oriented system to a rationalized bureaucracy. These shifts, in turn, have an important bearing on the psychological meaning of the doctor-patient relationship, on the uses of medical excuses for various social purposes, and on the flexibility of medicine as an institution to meet patient expectations and to relieve tensions in the community at large. The remainder of this paper will explicate each of these points.

Types of Rationing

In the traditional practice of medicine, and in much of the world still today, the availability of medical care has been dependent on the ability to purchase it. Those with means could obtain whatever level of medical care was available, while those without means were dependent on whatever services were made available by government, philanthropists, the church, or by physicians themselves. Since affluence was limited, and medical technology and knowledge in any case offered only modest gains, the marketplace was a natural device for rationing services. Indeed, it worked so well that physicians were often supporters of government intervention and direct payments for care since such support increased their opportunities for remuneration.

Fee-for-service as an effective system of rationing broke down due to a variety of factors. First, medical technology and knowledge expanded rapidly, greatly increasing the costs of a serious medical episode, and imposed on the ill a financial burden that was large and unpredictable. Associated with this was a growing demand on the part of the public for means of sharing such risks through benevolent societies and insurance plans and, as costs mounted, for government to assume a growing proportion of these expenditures. Because of the traditions of medical practice, however, and the political monopoly that physicians had gained over the marketplace, the rise of third-party payment was not associated with careful controls over the work of the physician and how he generated costs. While third-party payment increased access to services, the orientations of increasingly scientific and technologically inclined physicians resulted in a large acceleration in the use of diagnostic and treatment techniques. The consequence has been the escalation of costs which we now almost view as inevitable. Physicians have been trained to pursue the "technological imperative"—that is, the tendency to use any intervention possible regardless of cost if there is any possibility of gain (Fuchs, 1968). This contrasts with a cost-benefit calculation in which there is consideration of the relative costs and benefits of pursuing a particular course of action. The "technological imperative," when carried to its extreme, incurs fantastic expense for relatively small and, at times, counterproductive outcomes.

In a provocative analysis, Victor Fuchs (1976) asks why almost all the developed countries in the world pursue national health insurance when such a policy is "irrational" from an economic point of view in that it encourages the overconsumption of services relative to other needs. Moreover, he argues, it often results in the purchase of the wrong and, perhaps, less useful types of care. He comes up with the intriguing suggestion that the thrust toward national health insurance may have relatively little to do with health.

> Externalities, egalitarianism, the decline of the family and traditional religion, the need for national symbols—these all play a part. In democratic countries with homogeneous populations, people seem to want to take care of one another through programs such as national health insurance, as members of the same family do, although not to the same degree. In autocratic countries with heterogeneous populations, national health insurance is often imposed from above, partly as a device for strengthening national unity. The relative importance of different factors undoubtedly varies from country to country and time to time, but the fact that national health insurance can be viewed as serving so many diverse interests and needs is probably the best answer to why Bismarck and Woodcock are not such strange bedfellows after all.

Many developed nations shifted quite early away from fee-for-service rationing to what I have referred to as *implicit rationing*. Under health insurance plans in various European countries, rationing was imposed either by the centralized prospective budgeting procedures of the government, as in England, or through the limited resources available to "sickness societies" that contracted with physicians and hospitals for services for their members. For example, in England under the National Health Insurance Act of 1911, and later through the enactment of the National Health Service in 1946, the central government budgeted fixed amounts for providing community medical services on a capitation basis, and hospital services as of 1948 on a global budget. Similarly, "sickness societies" in other countries had to make contractual agreements with physicians within the means available, thus limiting the extent of services that could be rendered.

In European countries that adopted national health insurance through an indirect method, such as mandated employer-employee contributions, governments increasingly assumed a larger proportion of the costs of physician services and institutional care. Since government had little control over how costs were generated by physicians and hospitals, there was continuing pressure for increased expenditures by both patients and physicians. Governments took on the obligation in making up deficits between costs generated by health professionals and the funds available from employer-employee contributions. They did so either by raising the social security tax rates or by making larger contributions each year from general revenues. In England, where the government had direct budgetary control, costs were more successfully contained, but there were constant pressures from health professionals for increased expenditure, nevertheless. Despite direct control, the proportion of national income allocated to health care escalated, but at a lesser rate than in many other countries that had more open-ended budgeting systems.

Implicit rationing depends on the queue. Limited resources, facilities, and manpower are made available, and the health care system adapts to demand by establishing noneconomic barriers (Mechanic, 1976: 87–97). Health professionals, having their own styles of work and professional norms, accommodate as many patients as they can, making judgments as to priorities and need. Access to services may be limited by long appointment or referral waiting periods, by limited sites of care (and therefore greater barriers of distance and inconvenience), longer waiting times, bureaucratic barriers, and the like. Rationing also may occur through the control exercised over the extent of elaboration of services: the laboratory tests ordered, the diagnostic techniques used, the rate of hospitalization, the number of surgical interventions, and the time devoted to each patient. Capitation or salary as a form of professional payment tends to limit the extent of these modalities; fee-for-service increases the rate of discrete technical services for which a fee is paid (Glaser, 1970; Roemer, 1962).

Implicit rationing has the effect of limiting expenditures, but not necessarily in a rational way. Such rationing is based on the assumption that the professional is sufficiently programmed by his socialization as a health practitioner to make scientifically valid judgments as to what constitutes need, what treatment modalities are most likely to be effective, and which cases deserve priority. It is supposed that the exercise of clinical judgment will result in rational decision making. But as Eliot Freidson (1976:136–137) has noted, evaluation of medical judgment by professional peers is so permissive that only "blatant acts of ignorance or inattention" are clearly recognized as mistakes. Moreover, it is the more knowledgeable, more aggressive, and more demanding individuals who get more service; and these patients are usually more educated, more sophisticated, but less needy (Hetherington et al., 1975). In short, under implicit rationing the assumption is that physicians exercise agreed-upon standards for care and that services are equitably provided in light of these standards. The fact is that these standards are very murky, if they exist at all, and even the most obvious ones have little relationship to any existing knowledge on the implications of varying patterns of care for patient outcome. Under these conditions, the most effective and vocal consumers may get more than their share of whatever care is available. Moreover, given the ambiguities of practice, physicians and other health professionals may play out their own personal agendas, cultural preferences, and professional biases. Being remunerated on salary, they may work at a comfortable and leisurely pace; and they may choose to emphasize work they find most interesting, neglecting important needs of patients, such as needs for empathy and support, which may be perceived as professionally less fulfilling functions.

There is considerable evidence that systems of implicit rationing provide care at lower cost because of the limited budget available and the containment in provision of resources and manpower, but there is little evidence to support the contention that the result is a fairer allocation of social resources. Under implicit rationing, large disparities continue in the availability of facilities, in allocation of manpower and resources per capita (and in relation to known rates of morbidity in the population), and in access to services (Cooper, 1975; Logan, 1971; Hetherington et al., 1975). Affluent areas tend to retain more facilities, manpower, and other resources, and relatively little redistribution takes place. There are very large variations from area to area and institution to institution in the procedures performed, work load, ancillary assistance available, and the level of technology.

Increasingly, governments are seeking means to move from implicit to explicit forms of rationing. The idea of explicit rationing is not only to set limits on total expenditures for care, but also to develop mechanisms to arrive at more rational decisions as to relative investments in different areas of care, varying types of facilities and manpower, new technological initiatives, and the establishment of certain minimal uniform standards. The difficulty with establishing such priorities and standards is the overall lack of definitive evidence as to which health care practices really make a difference in illness outcomes. While standards for processes of care are readily formulated, it is difficult to demonstrate for most facets of care that such process norms have any clear relationship to outcomes that really matter. Indeed, health services random trials tend to show that such expensive innovations as coronary intensive care or longer hospitalizations for a variety of diseases seem to make little difference in measurable outcomes for populations where they are routinely used (Cochrane, 1972).

The difficulty of imposing explicit rationing, however, is more political than scientific. While there is always danger in establishing general guidelines that the overall formulation will not fit a specific case, there are many instances in medical practice where intelligent restrictions on practices of physicians are likely to lead to both improved and more economical practice. The fact is, however, that physicians resist such guidelines as intrusions on their professional judgment and autonomy, and tend to do whatever they can to subvert them. Even with a certain amount of slack, intelligent guidelines—sensitive to the realities of medical practice and human behavior—can be an important contribution toward more effective rationing than usually exists under the implicit system.

There are a variety of techniques that are used under many insurance systems to restrict the options of health practitioners (Glaser, 1970), and these are becoming more commonly adopted. The most straightforward is the simple exclusion or restriction of certain types of services that may involve large costs but dubious benefits—for example, psychoanalysis, orthodontia, rest cures, plastic surgery for cosmetic purposes, etc. In the case of essential components of treatment, the program may set maximal numbers of procedures that will be paid for or establish required time intervals between procedures that can be repeated and remain eligible for coverage. These limitations have the function of restricting the physician's discretion although to a modest degree. In theory, however, they can be very much extended. Another technique is to limit the cost of a treatment by requiring the physician to provide justification if he wishes to exercise a more expensive option. Since physicians tend to dislike additional required paperwork, if the guidelines are reasonable they are likely to be effective.

In the United States, emphasis is now being given to mandatory peer review, a process whereby utilization practices and, in the future, the quality of care as well will be evaluated. Moreover, justification under federal programs must be provided if certain established norms are to be exceeded. While these requirements are still very weak, and frequently insufficiently responsive to contingencies at the service level, and involve a great deal of unnecessary administrative effort, in theory they can be quite valuable if the review process is an intelligent one and if control over the review mechanism is not captured by physicians who wish to maintain ongoing practices. The necessity of any guideline or standard should be evaluated in terms of its costs and benefits. When the costs exceed the benefits, the rule is obviously pointless.

Some countries require pre-review for specified expensive procedures.

If pre-review is used too extensively it becomes a costly and inefficient technique but, if used sparingly to control expensive work of dubious effectiveness and possibly dangerous as well, it can have effects both as a deterrent and as a means of controlling irresponsible practitioners. Particularly in the area of surgical intervention and perhaps also in the use of dangerous classes of drugs, pre-review functions both to reduce costs and to encourage a higher quality of care. In short, both government itself and nongovernmental insurance programs are becoming more bold in intruding on areas that physicians regard as within their discretion. We have every reason to anticipate that this trend will continue.

Rationing and Primary Medical Care

The most salient aspect of medical organization in modern countries is the enormous growth of specialization and subspecialization that has occurred. While much of this development is due to the growth of biomedical science and technology, specialization is also a political process bringing economic advantages and greater control over one's work and responsibilities (Stevens, 1971). Specialization, moreover, allows physicians to dominate a specified domain and to restrict competition. While the traditional concept of the specialist was as a consultant physician who assisted the generalist with puzzling problems or those of greater complexity, existing specialties are organized around varying population groups such as pediatrics or geriatrics, types of technology such as radiology, organ systems such as nephrology, etiologies such as infectious disease, and disease categories such as pulmonary disease. The most recent distortion of the concept of the consulting physician was the development of a specialty in family practice, which in effect defines the generalist as another type of specialist.

While there are many issues relevant to the manner in which specialization has emerged, the distinction with the greatest importance for rationing is the one between physicians who engage in primary care and those who provide specialty care or more complex hospital services. Everywhere in the world, nations are seeking to define the appropriate functions and responsibilities for each of the levels of care and their most efficient balance. Most discussions of primary care, particularly in countries that retain the provision of services at least in part within the private marketplace, suffer from confusions among the organizational, service, and manpower dimensions of the situation.

The most typical view of primary care is that it is the care given by certain types of practitioners who work as generalists: general practitioners, family practitioners, nurse practitioners, and so on. It is assumed that the training received by such practitioners prepares them adequately to provide first-contact care and to take continuing responsibilities for overall needs of the patient. While convenient, this definition includes as primary care highly complex medical and surgical procedures that are more adequately performed by physicians who are highly conversant with the field and who perform these procedures sufficiently frequently to do them expertly. While a considerable amount of major surgery has been performed by general practitioners in the United States and elsewhere, major surgery is not appropriately included as primary care. Similarly, many specialists insist that they devote significant amounts of their time to primary care, and thus the shortage of primary care physicians is exaggerated. It should be clear then that this approach to understanding the appropriate role of primary care is not particularly helpful.

It is frequently suggested that one way of resolving the issue of primary care is to divide arbitrarily medical functions into primary, secondary, and tertiary. Such an approach, however, misses the major point which is that the practice of medicine is a conceptual and intellectual endeavor in which physicians with diverse training perceive, evaluate, classify, and manage comparable patients differently. The evaluation of a patient in good medical practice comes from listening to the patient, getting to know the person, and developing a clinical context in which the patient is willing to reveal himself or herself. How physicians will come to view a patient's problem depends on their orientations and how accessible the patient is to them psychologically as well as physically. The key point is that differences between primary and specialist practitioners are not simply a matter of what they do, but also a matter of how they do it. An essential aspect of primary care is the physician's attitude, assumptions and storage of information about the particular patient, and the way the practitioner goes about evaluating the patient's complaint. Many patients first contacting a physician are in a stage in which their symptoms are unorganized and fluid (Balint, 1957). What the physician defines as important, what he inquires about, and how he evaluates the patient's symptoms and illness behavior are molded by his knowledge of the patient as well as his training and orientations. In understanding how varying types of general and subspecialty training affect medical practice, it is necessary to have a good appreciation of how patients with comparable presenting complaints are evaluated and managed differently.

Still another way of viewing primary care is as part of an organizational system. Here the emphasis is less on a particular type of practitioner and how he is trained, and more on how different levels of care are organized and how they relate to one another. For example, in most organized medical care systems there are designated primary care physicians who have responsibility for first-contact care, for assuming continued responsibility for an enrolled population, and for dealing with the more common and less complicated problems of their patients. These systems are often established so that patients are required to seek more specialized services through the referral of their primary doctor. Similarly, secondary and tertiary care facilities are organized in relation to the system as a whole, and attempts are made to specify the conditions for coordination among varying levels of care. Although the particular type of practitioner used at varying levels of care is not an unimportant issue, the major focus shifts to defining responsibilities for care functions at each level of care. Primary care services, however they are defined by the system, may be organized in a variety of ways with alternative types of personnel as long as the necessary functions are performed. In this context, primary care is a level of service, not a particular type of practitioner.

The formulation of a planned system of primary, secondary, and tertiary functions has important implications for rationing. When the primary practitioner is the source of entry into the care system and a gatekeeper to access to more specialized practitioners and technologies, the rate of use of specialized technologies can be very much diminished. Systems of care that use primarily a sole source of entry through a primary physician make do with many fewer specialists and specialized facilities, and without any major loss in effective care. As Paul Beeson (1974:48), who has held responsible positions in both England and the United States, has noted:

> There are 22,000 in family practice in the United Kingdom and 70,000 in family practice in the United States. There are 8,000 in specialist practice in the United Kingdom and 280,000 in specialist practice in the United States. . . . The striking difference is economy in the use of specialists. To me this is the most obvious reason why America has a badly distributed, excessively costly system.

An effective system of care, moreover, allows an opportunity to organize manpower rationally relative to population groups, thus limiting the extent to which doctors generate marginal efforts due to their excessive concentration in any area. Also, by emphasizing functions and patterns of care, rather than types of medical specialties, it is much less difficult to develop functional substitutes to physicians in performing many primary care services. Because the emphasis is on a service, it is more possible to develop participation of health practitioners who are trained and willing to perform functions that physicians are unwilling to do, that they do poorly, or that they provide inefficiently—for example, health education, patient monitoring, medically related social services, and the like.

When primary care is defined as part of a system, problems still remain in coordination and motivation. The point at which referrals should take place from one level to another, for example, is left to the individual practitioner and is often affected by the implicit incentives built into the organization of health services or in how health personnel are remunerated. A common complaint in organized systems of care based on a capitation arrangement is that unnecessary referral is made to secondary services because of the lack of incentive for continued care at the primary level (Forsyth and Logan, 1968). These problems can be alleviated, if not avoided, by a good understanding of the epidemiology of help-seeking, with specification of standards for referral and with incentives promoting good care.

The Structure of Doctor-Patient Interaction
under Varying Rationing Arrangements

Each of the types of rationing described tends to be associated with a particular mode of physician-patient interaction, although there is great variation within each type, dependent on the personalities of the actors involved, the work load and work flow, and the incentives operative in any particular situation. Eliot Freidson (1961, 1970, 1976) has written extensively on these types of relationships, and in this section I draw heavily on his work. Very simply, it is my contention that, as rationing varies from fee-for-service to implicit to explicit rationing, the types of influence shift from client control to colleague control to bureaucratic control. Similarly, the nuances in the physician's role shift from "entrepreneur" to "expert" to "official."

Freidson has convincingly illustrated how the shift from fee-for-service practice to prepaid group practice is accompanied by lesser flexibility and responsiveness of the physician. When the retention of the patient is no longer an economic issue for the physician, there is no need to "humor the patient" nor bend to the patient's wishes when they are contrary to the physician's best judgment. Freidson argues that in the prepaid situation colleagues are a more important reference group, and while the physician may be more inflexible he may practice a higher standard of medical care. The extent to which differences between fee-for-service and prepaid practice will exist depends greatly on the competition for patients existing in any practice area. As competition increases, physicians may be more willing to provide greater amenities to patients and to be flexible to their requests in order to retain their patronage. When the physician has more patients than he requires, there may be little client control even in the fee-for-service situation. As the physician becomes less dependent on the patient—either because he is only one of a large number of physicians servicing an enrolled population or because he is in a favorable competitive situation—he can more easily play the role of the neutral expert, one whose decisions are quite isolated from any personal financial stake he may have in his work.

In theory, implicit rationing encourages the physician to play the role of the expert, but in actuality the difficulty lies in the ambiguity of his expertise. Since the physician by the very nature of his work is required to come to many social decisions quite irrelevant to his technical expertise, and since physicians differ radically on these social judgments, there is no clear basis for these decisions. For example, consider the frequently occurring issue of whether a hospitalized mother should be sent home or retained for a few more days because the physician anticipates that her family will expect her to resume usual duties, or because she may be inclined to quickly reassume responsibilities. In theory, when the patient must incur part of the fee, such potential cost will influence the decision. However, when third parties assume the cost, neither the physician nor the patient has any incentive to choose the more parsimonious decision. If the physician acts as an expert, his bias is to use resources if he sees any potential benefit. Incentives to do otherwise come only when he is personally faced with a limitation of resources. A global budget without further guidelines, although it may restrict the physician's actions to some extent, does not insure rational decision making and may encourage highly preferential behavior depending on the physician's perceptions of and attitudes toward the patient.

Although the evidence is not fully clear, most existing prepaid group practices seem to conserve resources more by controlling inputs—numbers of primary care physicians, beds, and specialists—than by directly affecting the manner in which physicians make decisions in allocating resources. While it has been alleged that the incentives for physicians to avoid unnecessary work may be an important factor, there is no impressive evidence that such incentives substantially affect decision making itself (Mechanic, 1976). Most of the rationing that takes place seems to be at the administrative planning level, and then physicians seem to adjust to whatever resources are available. Thus, in most prepaid group practices or in health centers or polyclinics, physicians still very much retain the role of "expert."

As health care plan administrators or government officials attempt to tighten expenditures by moving toward a system of explicit rationing, physicians are pushed to a larger degree into the role of bureaucratic official. The case of the Soviet physicians, described by Field (1957), who were limited in the number of sickness certifications they could issue, provides an extreme example of how bureaucratic regulation can substantially limit the options available for physician decision making. While no explicit rationing system in the world has gone this far in any systematic way, there is a discernible tendency toward greater administrative control. In such circumstances the physician must explicitly determine which patients are more needy of a particular service, and he must develop ways to discourage or influence other patients who insist on such service. Increasingly, for example, the physician will require pre-review of certain decisions or have other decisions reviewed after the fact. The intrusion of such requirements or review, if seriously performed, can have a significant effect on decision making, particularly on the "technological imperative."

Everywhere in the world physicians have retained considerable autonomy; even in such highly bureaucratized contexts as military medicine, industrial medicine, and the health services of communist countries, physicians have persisted in their roles more as experts than as bureaucratic functionaries. The shift is more nuance than drama, and while such tendencies will grow throughout the world, rationing is more likely to be imposed on the total framework of services and less on the decisions of the individual physician treating a particular patient. In any case, the growing bureaucratization of medicine poses some serious dangers, and I conclude this chapter with a brief consideration of these.

The Effects of Bureaucratization on Medicine as a Social Institution

Medicine as a social institution has extremely broad functions. Not only does medicine deal with the prevention and treatment of pain, disease, disability, and impairment, but it also provides an acceptable excuse for relief from ordinary obligations and responsibilities, and may be used to justify behaviors and interventions not ordinarily tolerated by the social system without significant sanctions. The definition of illness may also be used as a mechanism of social control to contain deviance, to remove misfits from particular social roles, or to encourage continued social functioning and productive activity. Thus, the locus of control for medical decision making is a key variable in examining the implications of medical care for social life more generally.

In the case of fee-for-service medicine, the physician acts as the agent of the patient. Although his own personal economic interests may intrude in the relationship, his role is to defend the interests of the patient against any other competing interest. The increasing employment of physicians by health programs or complex organizations involves changes in the auspices of medical care that depart in significant ways from traditional concepts (Mechanic, 1976). As I have noted throughout this paper, and specifically in my discussion of rationing, bureaucratic medical settings involve multiple interests, thus putting the physician under pressure to sacrifice certain potential interests of an individual patient to satisfy organizational needs. In the case of such institutions as health maintenance organizations, for example, increased administrative directions for rationing, as well as financial incentives, are developed to encourage physicians to avoid providing unnecessary services. But since the concept of "necessary" is itself vague, the determination may reflect the balance of pressures on the physician.

The bureaucratization of medicine also has the effect of diluting the personal responsibility of the provider, making it more likely that interests other than those of the patient will prevail. By segmenting responsibility for patient care, the medical bureaucracy relieves the physician of direct continuing responsibility. If the patient cannot reach a physician at night or on weekends, obtain responsive care, have inquiries answered, or whatever, the problem is no longer focused on the failure of an individual physician, but on the failures of the organization. It is far easier for patients to locate and deal with individual failures where responsibility is clear than to confront a diffuse organizational structure where responsibility is often hazy and the buck is easily passed. To the extent the physician knows that a patient is his or her charge, the physician feels a certain responsibility to protect the patient's interests against organizational roadblocks and requests that may not be fully appropriate. But when responsibility is less clear it is easier to make decisions in the name of other interests such as research, teaching, demonstration, or the "public welfare," whatever that might be.

The growth of bureaucratic medicine is in many ways an effective response to the development and complexity of medical knowledge. But it also involves some significant threats to the concept of physician responsibility for the best interests of the individual patient and for the empathic and supportive relationships that are so vital to effective care of the whole person. It also involves a shifting in the balance of power in dealing with the broader problems for which patients use the medical system such as in alleviating anxieties and excusing failure. The physician's role as advocate of the patient derives from a close and continuing relationship and knowledge of the patient and a certain relational alignment to him. Bureaucratic structures tend to promote more segmented and detached relationships and ambiguities and conflicts in relational alignments. While in theory bureaucratic structures could be developed to promote empathy, continuity, and humane care, the tendency is for bureaucratic and technical functions to be given higher priority. Physicians are rewarded more for being good managers and researchers or for coping with a large work load than for providing interested and humane care. While physician care in bureaucracies is often humane, such behavior seems to occur despite bureaucratic structure rather than because of it.

Bureaucratization in medicine is inevitable. The challenge thus is to promote organizational arrangements that ration wisely and fairly, and that provide incentives for listening to the patient and caring for him. Humane medicine is an effective component of good patient care. Medical outcomes often depend on the understanding and cooperation of patients and their willingness to engage their problems in a serious and committed way. Medicine without caring, no matter how effective the technique, has a limited capacity to fulfill the broad potential of medicine as a sustaining institution for those who come to depend upon it. The development of bureaucratic incentives, thus, must be designed to enhance humane values while capitalizing on advances in knowledge and technology (Howard and Strauss, 1975). In my estimation this can be most effectively accomplished by upgrading the role and performance of the primary care sector and by regulating carefully through the planning process the availability and provision of the more expensive, complex, and dangerous technologies. Within broad guidelines, physician and patient must remain as free as possible to negotiate satisfactory solutions to the personal and social dilemmas that bring them together.

References

Balint, Michael. 1957. *The Doctor, His Patient, and the Illness.* New York: International Universities Press.

Beeson, Paul. 1974. "Some good features of the British National Health Service." *Journal of Medical Education* 49 (January):43–49.

Cochrane, A. L. 1972. *Effectiveness and Efficiency: Random Reflections on Health Services.* London: Nuffield Provincial Hospitals Trust.

Cooper, Michael. 1975. *Rationing Health Care.* New York: John Wiley (Halsted Press).

Field, Mark. 1957. *Doctor and Patient in Soviet Russia.* Cambridge: Harvard University Press.

Forsyth, G., and Logan, R. 1968. *Gateway or Dividing Line: A Study of Hospital Out-Patients in the 1960's.* New York: Oxford University Press.

Fox, Renee, and Swazey, Judith. 1974. *The Courage to Fail: A Social View of Organ Transplants and Dialysis.* Chicago: University of Chicago Press.

Freidson, Eliot. 1961. *Patients' Views of Medical Practice.* New York: Russell Sage Foundation.

———. 1970. *Profession of Medicine: A Study of the Sociology of Applied Knowledge.* New York: Dodd-Mead.

———. 1976. *Doctoring Together: A Study of Professional Social Control.* New York: Elsevier.

Fuchs, Victor. 1968. "The growing demand for medical care." *New England Journal of Medicine* 279:190–195.

————. 1976. "From Bismarck to Woodcock: The 'irrational' pursuit of national health insurance." Center for Economic Analysis of Human Behavior and Social Institutions, Working Paper No. 120. National Bureau of Economic Research.

Glaser, William A. 1970. *Paying the Doctor: Systems of Remuneration and Their Effects*. Baltimore: Johns Hopkins Press.

Hetherington, Robert, et al. 1975. *Health Insurance Plans: Promise and Performance*. New York: Wiley-Interscience.

Howard, Jan, and Strauss, Anselm, eds. 1975. *Humanizing Health Care*. New York: Wiley-Interscience.

Logan, R. F. L. 1971. "National health planning—An appraisal of the state of the art." *International Journal of Health Services* 1 (February):6–17.

Mechanic, David. 1974. *Politics, Medicine, and Social Science*. New York: Wiley-Interscience.

————. 1976. *The Growth of Bureaucratic Medicine: An Inquiry into the Dynamics of Patient Behavior and the Organization of Medical Care*. New York: Wiley-Interscience.

Roemer, Milton. 1962. "On paying the doctor and the implications of different methods." *Journal of Health and Social Behavior* 3 (Spring):4–14.

Stevens, Rosemary. 1971. *American Medicine and the Public Interest*. New Haven: Yale University Press.

White, K. L., et al. 1961. "The ecology of medical care." *New England Journal of Medicine* 265:885–892.

2

Prospects and Problems in Health Services Research

Given the enormous growth of the health services field and the difficult problems associated with cost containment, regulation, quality assurance, and improvement of health behavior of the population, it might have been anticipated that health services research would be a growing and vigorous activity. Instead, the health services research field faces considerable skepticism among public officials and a significant erosion of its research and training support (National Research Council, 1977). Links between health services research and policy formulation and implementation are commonly challenged, and many leaders in government and the health care field are confused about the role and work of the health services research sector (Lewis, 1977). Improved understanding of the nature of health services research and its special problems will assist in developing realistic and appropriate criteria for public policies.

The health services research field focuses on the production, organization, distribution, and impact of services on health status, illness, and disability. Although the field shares certain concerns with behavioral studies, such as the determinants of health status, reactions to illness, health promotive behavior, and factors affecting adherence to medical advice, it concentrates attention on improving the distribution, quality, effectiveness, and efficiency of medical care. Because health services research is also often associated with demonstration projects and problems of technology transfer, these relationships require consideration despite the different emphases in demonstration and research programs.

Health services research involves activities similar in many respects to those carried out in the evaluation of educational, legal, or social welfare services. None of these other sectors, however, has expanded so rapidly or involves such complex forms of technology or social organization.

Research workers in the health services field come from a wider range of professional disciplines and educational backgrounds than researchers on education, law, or welfare, making interdisciplinary research and communication among research personnel more difficult. In short, although health services research is not a unique research field, it has special problems.

Vulnerability of the Health Services Research Sector

The health services research field is relatively young, having received major research support only in the last two decades (The President's Science Advisory Committee, 1972), and thus it is extremely vulnerable to instability in financing and uninformed criticism. Most other scientific activity is organized around disciplines with distinctive perspectives and professional organizations that serve as a basis for identification and effective lobbying. In contrast, health services research is carried out by members of a variety of disciplines such as physicians, sociologists, epidemiologists, biostatisticians, economists, or operations researchers. Although shared research concerns bring these professionals together, they have no clear organizational affiliation or professional identification around the health services research area. Most such researchers identify with their primary discipline, making it difficult to measure the research manpower available or even the boundaries of the field (National Research Council, 1977). Moreover, unlike the various interest groups representing the study of such diseases as cancer, heart disease, and mental illness, or highly organized disciplinary groups, such as biochemists or psychologists who maintain staff to promote their disciplinary involvements, health services research has no organized constituency to promote it.* Because health services research lacks the emotional appeal of categorical disease problems or the professional organization of traditional disciplines, support for the field must rest solely on its merits and potential. In this respect, the field continues to be handicapped by unrealistic expectations, inflated demands, and erratic modifications of its research agendas by funding agencies.

Although most basic research fields are oriented toward a particular community of scholars who share many assumptions, perspectives, and methodologies, health services research speaks more directly to policy makers and administrators who typically face pressing practical problems. Not only must health services research achieve a level of scientific rigor satisfactory to other professionals who scrutinize its theories and research

---

*Approximately five years ago such a group—the Association for Health Services Research—was established.

efforts, but it must also pose issues in ways that appear reasonable to decision makers. Demands for scientific rigor from one's colleagues often interfere with meeting the expectations of simplicity, comprehensibility, and need from the policy makers. One never hears complaints from administrators or legislators that research in immunology is worthless because they cannot understand it, but one frequently hears that health services research funding is being wasted on "incomprehensible regression equations." Thus, health services research faces not only the usual needs of a research discipline, but also the additional expectation of suitable translation.

Role of Health Services Research

The health services research effort is miniscule relative to the magnitude of the industry it scrutinizes, the intellectual scope of the problems it deals with, and the social and political context in which it must operate. Such research commonly deals with problems that involve strong ideologies, competing perspectives, and contending interests. Often the solutions desired are not simply technical and scientific but also decisions about values, and yet health services researchers are frequently admonished because they do not state clearly and unequivocally what should be done. Although administrators are not so naive as to anticipate that health services research can resolve political disputes, some administrators find health services research a convenient scapegoat when they feel frustrated by the difficulties of modifying the health care arena in any fundamental way.

The most serious problem affecting the future of health services research is the expectation that a modest research investment will provide solutions to the political dilemmas of health care. It is both naive and counterproductive to anticipate any direct relationship between such research and policy implementation. The demand that health services research questions be formulated in terms of immediate political issues, moreover, debases the processes of problem formulation, compromises adequate data acquisition, and inevitably leads to disappointment and frustration. To the extent that policy decisions are important, highly visible, and affect important contending interests, they depend more on political compromise than on particular research projects, although research results may help indirectly to inform the debate and shape the outcome. Although legislators may ask what research project ever led to a specific policy decision, the implication being that such research is of little value and unworthy of support, the fact is that the question is itself based on false and unrealistic premises. Health services research will (and, indeed, should) always be in the background in the formulation of important policy decisions unless the decisions are purely technical ones. But few important health services issues are simply matters of knowledge or technical expertise.

Health services research cannot solve the big policy issues, but it can perform a wide variety of functions including acquisition of descriptive information on the performance of the health services, analytic research and hypothesis testing on microissues, such as the effects of cost sharing on consumers or variations in remuneration on professionals, and evaluation of large sociomedical programs. It also is allied closely with demonstration programs in which the emphasis is less on theory and more on the practical issues of implementation and the diffusion of innovations. The major role of health services research is to inform the policy makers and implementers, but not determine their decisions or actions, although there are occasional exceptions on largely technical or apolitical matters. Through various kinds of health services research, issues are raised, observations made, and perspectives developed that over the long term affect the way administrators and politicians see problems, formulate options and approaches, and implement decisions. To the extent that health services research is done well, it contributes immensely to intelligent policy consideration and more than repays its relatively small investment. Unless we take a fairly long-range perspective, we may readily miss the extent to which our conceptions of health care problems have changed in the past decade or two, in large part because of health services research.

Although 20 years ago most observers had implicit faith that greater investments in health services would significantly improve the health of the nation, they now have much greater skepticism that larger health care investments bring commensurate results (Knowles, 1977). We are much more aware that the health status of the nation depends on environmental conditions and patterns of behavior outside the health care delivery system. We increasingly realize that the resources available, such as hospital beds, surgical specialists, and primary care physicians, affect the magnitude of demand and utilization and that there is an uncertain relationship between the use of more services and health status (Fuchs, 1974). We have learned to see that providing physician and other services is not simply an issue of numbers but also of distribution, and we are targeting our policies more specifically on the basis of such knowledge (Lewis, Fein, and Mechanic, 1976). We have learned a great deal about the benefits and problems of Health Maintenance Organizations (HMOs) and the ways they compare with alternative delivery systems, and of new personnel and facilities, such as physician assistants, nurse practitioners, perinatal units, and surgicenters. We are better informed of the imperfections of the medical marketplace and ways to deal with them, and of the relationship between financing and the manner in which services are produced. Although this may now seem to be the conventional wisdom of today, much of the way we see and do things is influenced by previous results of health services research.

Unlike research in most other disciplines, successful health services research attracts critics. Although we all applaud research developments in cancer, schizophrenia, or kidney disease, research on the performance of the health sector is frequently politically costly to particular professional groups. Surgeons hardly like the suggestion that they perform unnecessary surgery; hospitals dislike the implication that they are inefficient and wasteful; physicians recoil at suggestions that they create their own demand, offer ineffective care, and maintain political control over the medical marketplace. One hardly expects these groups to serve as a constituency in support of health services research.

The fact is, however, that a well-structured health services research program is essential to future health care policy and to adequate monitoring of a massive national investment. Almost every recent major piece of health legislation poses requirements for data acquisition, planning, and evaluation for which we lack the resources and often the theoretical and methodological sophistication as well. Questions posed quite glibly in political debate are often difficult to translate into scientific hypotheses that can be examined in any reasonable fashion. Although it is natural for those who want immediate answers to be impatient, many of the questions raised are complex and difficult, requiring long-term conceptual and empirical efforts. These considerations should make it clear that health services research is much more likely to contribute successfully if its concerns are more long term than short, and if its efforts can be separated from the immediate pressing needs of policy makers and administrators; health services research offers guidance and perspectives to policymakers who may not benefit in any immediate sense from health services research findings. With these considerations in mind, the functions of health services research are considered below, together with their relevance to research on other institutional sectors such as education, welfare, or law.

Information and Intelligence

One of the most acute needs of administrators is simply to know the facts: facts concerning gaps in the distribution of services; actual costs for medical and surgical procedures in varying localities; relationships between expenditures and changes in health status; rates of admission to hospitals and lengths of stay for varying procedures, and ways they are changing; costs of new technologies and how they affect physician behavior and medical outcomes; and many more. Moreover, administrators require some indication of impending problems both to formulate responses and to deal with possible political contingencies. Although we know a great deal about the performance of health services, we still lack many crucial facts despite their importance for future planning. Many such efforts to gather important facts routinely or on a periodic basis are made through the National Center for Health Statistics and a variety of special surveys carried out by health services researchers in universities. For example, the Center for Health Services Administration at the University of Chicago has carried out periodic surveys of national samples involving such issues as access to and expenditures for medical care. These surveys have provided data on trends that allow assessment of the progress made in such areas as extending access. University researchers carry out survey studies on such varied issues as health and illness behavior, utilization of care, physician attitudes, adjustment of the handicapped, and the social needs of the aged.

Acquiring facts is not simple because they depend on concepts that may be unclear or difficult to measure. What is the meaning of a physician visit when the content of such visits varies widely from one context to another and includes office visits and phone visits? How does one estimate the prevalence of psychiatric disorder when experts disagree on appropriate definitions? How does one measure the impact of medical care on health status when we lack valid and reliable measures of the dependent variable? How do we estimate the total expenditures for physician services when some of these expenditures are included in hospital charges? Behind many simple facts are serious problems of concept and methodology that continue to require considerable developmental efforts if we are to generate reliable information for sound decision making.

In addition to routine monitoring through large-scale surveys and statistical reporting systems, we need more detailed information on how the epidemiology of disease is changing in the community; the types of case mix seen in varying types of facilities; the procedures and costs generated by varying types of medical encounters; and the impact of changing patterns of professional work, new technologies, and innovative facilities. What, for example, are the case-fatality rates for varying types of medical and surgical procedures in varying types of facilities? Are physicians typically doing more laboratory procedures in routine medical examinations and do they vary by type of specialty, organizational setting, or type of patient? What is the fate of patients released from institutions as part of the emphasis on deinstitutionalization programs? What services are they receiving, what problems are they having, and what is their level of functioning in varying types of community settings? Although it is difficult to anticipate which of the many descriptive questions concerning health services will become special agenda items for policy makers, continuing descriptive efforts both contribute to the anticipation of impending problems and provide a data base from which to begin to formulate political options.

Analytic Research and Hypothesis Testing

Health services research also includes more complex studies that may not have immediate relevance but contribute in a general way to informing policy makers. Such studies generally involve testing hypotheses about the impacts of various types of incentives and other interventions. Such studies might include hypotheses about the effects of coinsurance and deductibles on rates of utilization, on the impact of remunerating physicians by capitation or salary in contrast to fee for service, and on the performance of nurse practitioners as compared with physicians. Such studies also vary in their concerns and may reflect the state of current knowledge, the ingenuity of the investigator, the variations present in the health care system, the possibilities of initiating new programs and experiments, and the limits of research personnel and funding. Although in the long run many of these studies will not be particularly useful to the policy maker, they make up the intellectual resources of the health services field and serve as the basis for new ideas. Thus, investments in health services research must be seen in a probabilistic sense; it is essential to fund a broad range of studies to generate those that will be important in affecting thinking and future efforts. As with biomedical research, it is necessary to explore many paths, knowing that some will be *cul-de-sacs*.

Although administrators can define certain areas of present interest, there is no effective way of targeting such knowledge-building efforts. A modest but stable research program is needed to facilitate the work of academic researchers who generate ideas based on their own theories, observations, and experience. Certainly, a field as large as health services can afford this risk capital to insure that at least some segment of research goes beyond the current notions of what is relevant and practical.

Evaluation Research

Another health services research effort involves evaluation of new and ongoing programs. These studies are particularly difficult and frequently disappointing because many do not have clearly defined or agreed upon goals. Often, the coalition necessary to put a program together involves groups with varying goals and definitions, yet maintaining a vague symbolic definition of the program's purpose serves important political needs. No one may really expect the program to have the impact suggested by political rhetoric, and it may be pointless to study whether it really does. Other barriers to evaluation include the reluctance of administrators to risk a negative assessment; the tendency to modify programs repeatedly before an evaluation is completed, thus complicating and undermining the evaluation; and a variety of methodological problems inherent in any complex evaluative effort.

To the extent that the evaluator views his task as comparable to a controlled clinical trial, he faces a high likelihood of failure. Most important evaluations performed from outside an ongoing system tend to get caught in a critical cross fire from those who have something to lose, and there are innumerable opportunities to sabotage any such data collection. Evaluations that are seen as attempts to improve practice through identifying problems and unexpected consequences—and that are organized in close cooperation with those who execute programs—have more potential. Most professionals are open to improving their practices if they are not threatened, and thus the challenge in evaluation is to provide productive feedback without arousing defensiveness.

Evaluations as experiments are more viable when there are no large organizational repercussions resulting from the outcome, when they are unlikely to identify particular organizations as having failed, and when they address relatively discrete analytical questions. Evaluations are usually poorly received when they involve one specific program or agency, when the goals of the program are relatively ambiguous, and when the organization is at political risk. Thus, large-scale experimental evaluations are more feasible for examining the impact of different insurance programs or the effect of providing income grants on willingness to work than they are in examining the effectiveness of community mental health centers or biomedical training programs.

In the health services field we need a great deal of formative evaluation that provides feedback to programmatic personnel as to the impact of their efforts, unexpected consequences, and the way administrative principles are being translated at the grass roots level. Thus, evaluation becomes part of an iterative process in which the evaluator becomes one more member of the program team rather than an outside observer grading its performance.

Policy Analysis

Policy analysis applies social and economic analytical techniques and existing data for the purpose of suggesting the costs and benefits of particular policy initiatives. Such analysis involves understanding not only the substance of the problem to be attacked but also the policy-making process and the realistic possibilities and constraints of government. Because policy analysis is so closely allied with the political process, much of it must be performed within the context of an ongoing governmental process. Although an outside policy analyst might suggest new policy options or provide useful technical advice, all policy suggestions go through a continuous process of review and modification before being used, and only by close contact is it possible to perform an effective role in implementation.

Government administrators, however, must react to continuing demands of an immediate nature. Thus, their focus is relatively short range, and their energies and attentions tend to be devoted to the issues of the moment. Long-range analysis is needed, however, to examine policy questions thoroughly, compare alternative options and their cost and benefits, and consider the processes of implementation and the ways they might be achieved under existing restraints. Such activity requires a certain separation from the day-to-day efforts of government but with enough communication to insure consistency with political and administrative realities.

Demonstration and Diffusion

Tasks of demonstration and technology transfer are quite different from those of health services research, but such efforts can gain from health services research as well as providing a laboratory in which to study difficult problems of implementation and diffusion of new knowledge and techniques. The health system is characterized by considerable diversity and diffusion of responsibility and the decision making. There is a complex—and often circuitous—path between demonstrating that something can work and making it work in varied settings that may lack the leadership, motivation, momentum, or supervision that existed at the demonstration site. Every new demonstration, like the introduction of new drugs, may have an impact associated with the expectations and enthusiasm it generates. If a new technology or organizational arrangement is to be effective, however, it must work in the ordinary situation and maintain its impact over time. Problems of the transfer of knowledge, technology, and social organization include problems of leadership, motivation, incentives, skills, and attitudes, and intimately involve the culture of institutions. They constitute perhaps the most difficult and problematic area in the entire health services arena.

The transfer of health services organizational arrangements, as in the development of HMOs, has many of the same problems as the transfer of biomedical knowledge and technology, but it is infinitely more complex in a political and sociological sense. In the case of the transfer of biomedical technologies, such as new drugs or CAT scanners, there may be no major organizational changes required, and the adoption of the innovation may be consistent with existing ideological and economic interests. There still remains the problem, however, of teaching large dispersed populations of physicians to use the technology wisely and when indicated. Although new technologies may be adopted quickly, they may be used inappropriately, as in the prescription of antibiotics. However, when organizational innovations are at issue, they more commonly require fundamental modifications in professional alignments and routines, and may threaten the roles, statuses, and economic security of particular individuals or groups. Thus, it is much easier for physicians to accept a new drug or a new diagnostic practice than to introduce a nurse practitioner into their practice or a change in any fundamental way in which they relate to patients. The fact that Kaiser can organize HMOs that perform reasonably well is no assurance that other organizations lacking similar histories, ideological commitments, leadership, and experience can achieve the same outcomes.

The problems associated with transfer of innovations define a large agenda of needed health services research. Because conditions vary from one setting to another, it is essential to replicate and monitor innovations in a variety of settings to identify the extent to which they differ in performance. Such replications are also necessary to reassure new adopters that the success of the innovation was not dependent solely on the special skills of those who initiated it, but that the idea is adaptable to settings like their own. Repeated studies of nurse practitioner deployment, for example, build a momentum that breaks down barriers to the use of such personnel among physicians who come to feel more secure in trying new approaches once they see others successfully doing so.

We need improved understanding of how to support innovations that tend to be fragile and easily undermined. The bind of traditional practice is very strong, and most organizational innovations either fail or take on more conventional coloration. Also, we need a better grasp of the factors that explain why some innovations diffuse rapidly while others that are successfully executed are never repeated. Although stable funding that allows an innovation to develop is a crucial factor, we need a more precise delineation of the incentives, cultural conditions, and technical support required to encourage more rapid deployment of useful innovations.

Conclusions

Administrators and policy makers are frequently impatient with health services research if it is not immediately relevant and practical. They question the value of research that does not directly result in policy implementation and that deals with more abstract theoretical and methodological issues. Health services research, however, has affected the climate of policy making, and its options are considered to a much larger degree than is generally recognized; health services research has achieved this more through long-range efforts and basic studies than through an emphasis on immediate practicality.

The fact is that the same basic issues and dilemmas in health care have persisted for years, suggesting that this is not due to a failure to focus on the practical but more to economic, political, ideological, and conceptual dilemmas that make it so difficult to reach an effective consensus. Although at any given point in time the administrator's options are limited, understanding problems in the long term sharpens policy thinking and contributes to successful policy formulation. Fundamental examination of questions dealing with cost containment, professional behavior, forces affecting health, consumer attitudes, and response within a broad context will suggest perspectives and options likely to inform the climate of future action. The health industry is enormous in size and complex in organization and increasingly faces difficult social, economic, and ethical dilemmas. Health services research is a tiny but valuable endeavor that provides a basic understanding of the way the health sector functions and its impact on the population. Maintaining and further developing such research activity are investments worthy of our attention and support.

References

1. National Research Council. 1977. *Personnel Needs and Training for Biomedical and Behavioral Research*. Volume 1, pp. 128–149. Washington, D.C.: National Academy of Sciences.
2. Lewis, C. E. 1977. Health-Services Research and Innovations in Health-Care Delivery: Does Research Make a Difference? *The New England Journal of Medicine* 297: 423–427.
3. The President's Science Advisory Committee. 1972. Improving Health Care Through Research and Development. *Report of the Panel on Health Services Research and Development*. Washington, D.C.: Executive Office of the President.
4. Knowles, J. (ed). 1977. Doing Better and Feeling Worse: Health in the United States. *Daedalus* 106 (winter): entire issue.
5. Fuchs, V. R. 1974. *Who Shall Live? Health, Economics, and Social Choice*. New York: Basic Books.
6. Lewis, C. E., Fein, R., and Mechanic, D. 1976. *A Right to Health: The Problem of Access to Primary Medical Care*. New York: Wiley-Interscience.

3

Policy Studies and Medical Care Research

Medical care or health services research, in contrast to biomedical research, has had modest discernible impact on public policy, the behavior of health professionals, or the organization of health facilities. Although it is possible to find instances where persons with official responsibilities justify particular policies through references to specific research, there is little evidence that the initiation of policy flows directly from research findings. Research, however, may in the long run help shape the climate within which decisions are made.

Part of the difficulty in discerning the impact of research on policy reflects the vagueness of the concept of policy itself. If by policy we mean legislative and governmental administrative actions, then it is obvious that research is only one of many relevant factors that are taken into account. At this level, it is clear that the range of variables that are seen as amenable to manipulation is limited at any point in time, and political feasibility is an important consideration. If we think of policy in terms of administrative actions at a variety of levels of organizational functioning, then we face a problem of diffusion of results. In a pluralistic system where there is a multitude of decision points, we would not expect that a solution demonstrated in one context would necessarily be seen as relevant or adaptable to another. Thus, solutions affecting smaller units of organization often diffuse very slowly, if at all. In considering the impact on policy, it is not apparent what criteria are reasonable to impose or what constitutes an appropriate span of time for diffusion to take place.

It may be that in the long run the most important impact of social research on policy results from the extent to which it affects the climate of thinking in the society at large. Research results and approaches diffuse in the media and have an effect on how educated persons think about problems. Policy-makers, like others, are affected by the climate of opinion in which they function, and research may have a crucial indirect role on how policy options are analyzed and how policy decisions are made and implemented.

Yet even in considering the diffusion process it is clear that some findings diffuse rapidly while others have little success. One can observe, for example, that findings in the area of biomedical technology and science have greater effectiveness than in most health services research. This is partly because the former tends to shape technology without intruding in major ways on the interests or life styles of professionals, while the latter poses greater threat to professional autonomy, work priorities, and control over work. In this chapter I will examine some of the difficulties in implementing health care research by focusing on studies dealing with social and psychological factors in the treatment of hospital patients and with the failure of physicians and medical facilities to give adequate attention to such concerns.

For the purposes of this chapter I will examine two studies carried out at Yale-New Haven (a Yale University teaching hospital): (1) a very specific experimental study of the role of communication in patient care; and (2) a general investigation of the quality of patient care. The first study (Skipper and Leonard 1968) rigorously performed and yielding specific results and implications for intervention, has been generally ignored. The second (Duff and Hollingshead 1968), a provocative descriptive study with both important implications but also serious methodological problems, resulted in a vigorous counter-attack by elite members of the academic medical establishment (Beeson 1968; Inglefinger 1968). I wish to discuss these works as part of a larger line of inquiry, since findings documenting the failure to give adequate attention to social and psychological factors are common in the literature (Cartwright 1964; Ley and Spelman 1967). It is my assessment that the rejection of the second study would have occurred regardless of its methodological rigor, since similar findings have been reported based on a variety of methodologies and these too have been ignored for the most part.

In the first study, reported by Skipper and Leonard, children admitted to a hospital for tonsillectomy were randomly divided into experimental and control groups. In the control group, patients received the usual care, whereas in the experimental situation, mothers were admitted to the hospital by a specially trained nurse who tried to facilitate communication and to maximize the mothers' opportunities to express their anxiety and to ask questions. An attempt was made to give the mother an accurate picture of the realities, and mothers were told what routine events to expect and when they were likely to occur. Mothers in the experimental group experienced less stress. Their children experienced smaller changes in blood pressure, temperature, and other physiological measures; they were less likely to suffer from post-hospital emesis and made a better adaptation to the hospital. These children made a more rapid recovery following hospitalization, displaying less fear, less crying, and less disturbed sleep than children in the control group. In considering this study, we note that tonsillectomy has been one of the most frequent surgical procedures performed in the United States, and the main cause of hospitalization of children (National Center for Health Statistics 1971). Controlled studies have demonstrated tonsillectomy to be a dubious surgical procedure in the great majority of cases, and psychological problems have been found to be a major adverse effect of the procedure, especially in young children. Thus, the importance of alleviating the distress of mother and child when the procedure is performed should not be minimized.

I have discussed the study with the investigators and various other persons associated with the hospital in which the study was carried out. There is consensus that the study had very little impact on the delivery of services. The innovation was not continued beyond the study period, and it had no observable effect on the general philosophy of patient care. It is likely that the results of the study at the hospital are not widely known, and there is agreement that the medical and surgical staffs have little interest in such studies. One of the investigators told me that a high-ranking physician on the staff asked him why he was wasting his time with such trivial problems.

The second study, carried out by Duff and Hollingshead, describes in some detail the general problems and complexity of a major teaching hospital, but focuses on a sample of 161 patients who received care on medical and surgical services in the private and ward facilities of the hospital. The investigators extensively interviewed patients, doctors, nurses, families, and other hospital personnel, examined medical records, observed patient care, and made follow-up visits to the patients when they returned home. Many of the findings are based on Duff and Hollingshead's global appraisal of each case and, except for anecdote, it is difficult to assess specifically how they made various judgments. Yet two major findings emerge from the study which I believe are unchallengeable, despite the fragility of the methodological approach. First, it is clear that a very different style of patient care prevails on the public in contrast to the private services, and that patients on the public wards were more likely to be taken for granted. Second, this study dramatically illustrates the failure of physicians to become sufficiently aware of their patients' social and psychological circumstances and to take these into consideration in the total management of these patients. Without accepting Duff and Hollingshead's specific evaluations of the adequacy of diagnosis, the mental status or adjustments of individual patients, or on many other technical matters, it is difficult for me to see how an impartial reader can reject the more general conclusion that there was a consistent failure to give adequate attention to the life circumstances of patients in relation to their illnesses. Nor is this observation inconsistent with observations elsewhere. The recommendations by Duff and Hollingshead are rather modest in relation to the magnitude of the issues they raise, but among them are such suggestions as "health professionals be trained to deal systematically with the personal and social factors which affect the diagnosis and treatment of patients [1968]."

Unlike many other investigators in the area, Duff and Hollingshead published their findings as a "trade" book, and it was accompanied by considerable newspaper publicity, including an article in *McCall's Magazine* (Pines 1968). Perhaps because of its public visibility it brought forth on the one hand criticism for failure to publish "results via accepted channels for scholarly communication" and on the other a public rebuttal in *Harper's Magazine* (Ingelfinger 1968).

The counterattack on Duff and Hollingshead came from two elite members of the academic establishment: Beeson (1968) of Oxford University, who had been chief of the Yale University Medical Service during the study period, and Ingelfinger (1968), editor of the *New England Journal of Medicine*. Both men, usually described as enlightened and progressive forces in medical care, offer a detailed rejoiner which at times borders on the petty. Both make an issue, for example, of the fact that Dr. Duff, an associate professor of pediatrics at Yale, described his interests in the preface of the book as "not exactly medicine and not necessarily sociology."

I do not believe that the methodological problems in the Duff-Hollingshead study were key issues in the rejection of the study since research findings on behavioral factors in disease have been generally ignored regardless of results, the type of study, or the rigors of methodology. Rigor and methodological adequacy are obviously important considerations, but it is striking how frequently weak and uncertain results are cited in support of one or another position when they support the viewpoint of the advocate. A dual standard seems to be imposed: one for studies whose findings you like, and quite another for those whose findings appear less attractive. This seems to be the case particularly when policy positions are advocated, and it supports the earlier observation that research results are used more frequently to justify policies than to suggest new approaches.

Although Duff and Hollingshead's attempt to make the issues public through the popular presentation and promotion of their book was bitterly criticized, they were at least able to elicit a hearing. Although the powers that be at Yale-New Haven were probably sufficiently angry with the results of the study to facilitate its rejection, and although the study had no apparent effect on the organization of services at the hospital, it has contributed importantly to discussions of the issues raised in the larger society and among younger health professionals. Thus, despite the study's lack of demonstrable, direct impact, it has probably generated a climate of concern. It is difficult to evaluate the effect of a "trade" book in contrast to journal articles in a particular case, but if *Science Citation Index* is any indication of the extent to which a particular project arouses interest in the scientific community, then it is clear that the Duff-Hollingshead study was considerably more successful than the Skipper-Leonard investigation. As one of the authors of the latter study wrote me in a response to an earlier draft of this paper, "accepted channels" may simply be a way of burying a study.

In considering why the Duff-Hollingshead study had little effect on the functioning of the Yale-New Haven hospital and why it would be unlikely to have effect regardless of its level of methodological elegance, I suggest that the implications of the findings are simply too radical. Such studies have little effect because, if taken seriously, they would require a fundamental reorganization of how medical services are delivered and how health personnel are trained. In this regard, Duff and Hollingshead show too little appreciation of the fundamental reorganization of medical education and practice necessary to achieve what they would like. Their limited specific recommendations, if implemented, would have very little effect in the face of the existing pattern of medical and hospital work.

It is therefore instructive to consider the larger criticisms of the Duff-Hollingshead study that are not specifically directed to their methodology or their motives. Such criticisms basically fall into two groups.

1. Both critics make the point that hospitals deal with serious organic disease and thus must establish priorities in terms of known interventions. They argue that since time and energy are limited, you do what you know how to do. As Ingelfinger puts it: " 'I rob banks,' said Willie Sutton, 'because that's where the money is.' "

2. Both critics deeply resent the unveiling of the "mystique of medicine." Both take bitter exception to what, as far as I can tell, is an accurate account of the process of obtaining autopsy permissions and of the methods used. This criticism tends to be an attack on sociology itself, since both critics imply that it was irresponsible to unmask the process. Ingelfinger describes this as "preoccupation with learning in its most ghoulish aspects," and Beeson makes the hysterical statement that "I'm sure that no lay person who has read their book will ever grant this

permission after the death of a relative.'' I cite this because both reviews, by men of unquestionable repute, display considerable paternalism in their discussions of patient care. They imply that patients have no right to know about the more ghoulish aspects of hospital care, since the mystique of medicine is truly in their interests.

Perhaps because Ingelfinger was less personally involved, he expresses greater ambivalence in his review and is more willing to concede that Duff and Hollingshead have raised important issues, although he criticizes their one-sided presentation of them. In respect to the difficult problem of weighing the need for further diagnostic search against the possibility that psychogenic factors are the cause of the patient's difficulty, he notes that ''There is no easy solution to the philosophical and moral problem, but to use this dilemma to 'prove' the narrow focus of the physician's interest or his lack of diagnostic drive verges on demagoguery [1968].''

Although Ingelfinger has probably overstated his point, he does raise a serious problem with the Duff-Hollingshead work and many other socio-logical studies in the "debunking" tradition. For the study is presented in terms of patient advocacy, and Duff and Hollingshead do not present the issues as seen by each of the major participants. In depicting the process of obtaining an autopsy and in its implications of disapproval of the means, it does not give attention to the high-minded ends that have produced such adaptations. And this is the crux of the issue. Both Ingelfinger and Beeson point out repeatedly the noble ends that have their associated seamy aspects, but Duff and Hollingshead chose to emphasize the seamy aspects and gave little attention to the noble ends. As Beeson notes in exaspera-tion: ''The authors' combination of smugness and naivete is hard to bear by someone who has been dealing with the realities [1968].''

I find the issue of autopsy a particularly interesting one since both Duff and Hollingshead and their critics miss or disregard what I regard as the crucial point. Clearly, autopsies are important for evaluation of work, continuing education, and improved performance; and any teaching hos-pital worthy of the name will attempt to obtain permissions to perform autopsies. In their zealousness, physicians sometimes commit the types of excesses described vividly in the Duff-Hollingshead volume and may even cajole and trick persons into providing the necessary permission. While Beeson and Ingelfinger focus on the noble functions of the autopsy, Duff and Hollingshead focus on the excesses. Neither examines how to balance the needs of the teaching hospital with the rights of patients and how their families are to be treated with dignity and be given a true opportunity to consent to requests. Achieving this is, of course, a complex and time-consuming process, and teaching hospitals are busy places. But when ends come to justify contemptible methods, we pay a price irrespective of the technical gains. Physicians also come to pay a price; for we are what we do, it may be argued, and the doctor who comes to adopt functional "tricks" loses some of his humanity.

In Beeson's view, "A low-keyed, well-documented report, aimed at professionals and written for professionals, could have immense and lasting value. After all, doctors and nurses are the only people who possibly can alter the conditions of patient care [1968]." This is in sharp contrast to the Duff-Hollingshead view that *"The answer is basically a society-wide issue rather than a problem for medical professionals alone.* Sickness is inextricably linked with society and society will have to look at itself for the solution [1968]." It is within these two contrasting views that the positions on both sides can be understood.

Beeson sees the solution to problems largely in terms of the efforts and good will of individual actors. He contends that since physicians and nurses provide care, change must come through influencing them to view some forms of professional behavior as desirable in relation to others. He appears to see sociological research in medicine as ancillary to the medical function, as one more aid to assist the physician and nurse to do a better job. In this light he views the Duff-Hollingshead book as a bitter and unjustified attack on medicine itself or, as Ingelfinger puts it, opening "new veins of muck for those who make it their business to rake the medical profession [1968]." In contrast, Duff and Hollingshead are indicting the structure of medical care itself and the societal pressures and values that sustain it in its present form. Although this attack on the basic structure of medical care in America is never fully or adequately developed, it seems apparent—although not to the physicians involved—that it is not a personal indictment. This is reflected in the following way. Duff and Hollingshead frequently quoted young physicians who from time to time used expressions among colleagues that they would be unlikely to use elsewhere; this is, of course, typical in the back regions of all occupations and may even be seen as a way of adapting to the stresses of work and uncertainty. Beeson, however, takes these anecdotes personally and views them as degrading:

> The criticism of the house staff extended even to attributing phrases to them which to me have a phoney ring, and perhaps merely represent what Duff and Hollingshead thought such characters ought to say! For example, I never heard the wards of the hospital referred to as "the zoo," nor do I think that the Emergency Admission Room was commonly referred to as "the pit." . . . I knew these young people well, far better than the writers of this book. I regarded them as able, likeable, dedicated and hard working—on the way to becoming outstandingly good physicians and surgeons [1968].

The basic issues of how to effectively utilize knowledge of patients' life situations in diagnosis, patient care, and rehabilitation, and how to weigh more elaborate attempts at physical diagnosis in contrast to considering other approaches to the patients' problems are difficult issues. We lack clear-cut concepts of how to appraise such difficulties or to effectively intervene, and it is natural that medical efforts should emphasize scientific medical orientations to care. However, in focusing on such problems, one risks a tendency of becoming callous and is likely to forget that medicine is a social art as well as a science. Moreover, the teaching hospital is the training ground not only for physicians who care for the desperately ill but for all physicians, and its emphases and orientations may not be well suited for much of the care physicians are called on to provide. In the care of even the seriously ill patient, social and psychological factors are of major importance; but the teaching hospitals have largely ignored these factors and thereby encouraged future generations of physicians to give them a low priority.

In conclusion, what can we learn from such controversies that may be helpful in making future efforts more effective? It is increasingly clear that if the intent of such studies is to bring about change in the contexts studied, rather than to add to knowledge or to inform the climate of general opinion, it is necessary to involve in such investigations those who have operational authority for the programs studied. In studying medical services, those concerned should be intimately involved in the design and progress of the study, and the investigation should require "informed consent" not only for the patients but also for the professionals involved. As a sociologist who works in medical contexts, I can attest to how difficult this can be. And, like the physician who fails to tell the patient everything in order to facilitate his management of the patient, the sociologist is also frequently tempted to say less than necessary in order to protect his access to the situation. I have increasingly come to believe that sociologists ought not to work on units in which the medical leadership will not accept them with a *realistic* understanding of the advantages and risks of sociological research. I emphasize the word "realistic" because it has been my experience that physicians who expect too much from behavioral science are as difficult to cooperate with as those who expect too little. It is crucial that physicians involved with behavioral science research programs in medicine have a reasonable concept of the likely product and the strengths and weaknesses of behavioral studies. It may be necessary in some contexts, such as in custodial institutions, to keep research concerns more covert, but it is unlikely to stimulate change from within. To the extent that the physicians are themselves involved in medical care research and committed to it, it is more likely that significant findings will be implemented.

It is also likely that research resulting in recommendations for fundamental restructuring of activities is unlikely to yield significant change. If Duff and Hollingshead were more analytic in their book, it would be clear that the failures of the teaching hospital cannot be resolved by simple changes here and there, but require substantial restructuring of health care financing, medical education, and medical practice. Professionals must work within the context of real constraints, and thus global recommendations for restructuring the overall approach leave helpless those who are urged to make the adaptations. In this sense Duff and Hollingshead were basically correct that the issues at stake are issues for the larger society and not just for the health professionals involved. In this sense the authors were using their observations at Yale-New Haven for a larger purpose, and their results have limited implications for reform of Yale-New Haven outside of more extensive reforms of the health care system as a whole. It is unfortunate that the study alienated some whose support will be needed in implementing the changes necessary to integrate social and psychological considerations in medical education and medical care. These differences, in part, represent conflicts of perspective that to some extent are inevitable; but they also suggest the importance of careful planning not only of the research effort, but also of the relationship of the researcher to the institutions studied.

References

Beeson, P.
    1968   Special book review of sickness and society, *Yale Journal of Biology and Medicine* 41, 226–240.
Cartwright, A.
    1964   *Human relations and hospital care*. Boston: Routledge and Kegan Paul.
Duff, R. S. and A. B. Hollingshead
    1968   *Sickness and society*. New York: Harper.
Ingelfinger, F. J.
    1968   The arch-hospital: An ailing monopoly, *Harper's Magazine:* 82–87.
Ley, P. and M. S. Spelman
    1967   *Communicating with the patient*. London: Trinity Press.
National Center for Health Statistics.
    1971   *Surgical operations in short-stay hospitals for discharged patients: United States—1965*. PHS Series 13, No. 7, April. Washington, D.C.: U.S. Government Printing Office.
Pines, M.
    1968   Hospital, *McCall's* 79, 138–142.

Skipper, J., Jr. and R. Leonard
  1968 Children, stress, and hospitalization: A field experiment, *Journal of Health and Social Behavior* 9, 275–287.

Part II
SOME GENERAL PERSPECTIVES
AND APPROACHES

4

The Concept of Illness Behaviour: Culture, Situation, and Personal Predisposition

The concept of illness or disease refers to limited scientific models for characterizing constellations of symptoms and the conditions underlying them. The concept of *illness behaviour,* in contrast, describes the ways in which people respond to bodily indications and the conditions under which they come to view them as abnormal. Illness behaviour thus involves the manner in which individuals monitor their bodies, define and interpret their symptoms, take remedial action, and utilize sources of help as well as the more formal health care system. It also is concerned with how people monitor and respond to symptoms and symptom change over the course of an illness and how this affects behaviour, remedial actions taken, and response to treatment. The different perceptions, evaluations and responses to illness have, at times, a dramatic impact on the extent to which symptoms interfere with usual life routines, chronicity, attainment of appropriate care and cooperation of the patient in treatment. Variables affecting illness behaviour usually come into play well before any medical scrutiny and treatment (Mechanic, 1978).

A crucial premise in the study of illness behaviour is that illness, as well as illness experience, is shaped by sociocultural and social-psychological factors, irrespective of their genetic, physiological or other biological bases. Away from the research laboratory, illness is often used to achieve a variety of social and personal objectives having little to do with biological systems or the pathogenesis of disease. The boundaries of illness and its definitions are potentially very broad, and the illness process can be used to negotiate a range of cultural, social and personal tensions in the home, at work, and in the community at large.

Cultural definitions, social development and personal needs shape the experience of illness and meanings attributed to physical factors that serve

59

as its basis. While the magnitude, severity, persistence and character of symptoms affect and establish limits for personal and social definitions, there is considerable variability in what is perceived, how it is defined, the interventions that are considered and used, requests for support and special consideration, and illness outcomes.

A major gap in our knowledge concerns those processes that lead persons exposed to similar stressors to respond differentially at a physical, psychological or social level. While the neuropsychological bases of alternative patterns of expressing distress remain uncertain, many research workers have ingeniously demonstrated that there may be conversions among different levels of experience and that substitutability among levels of response is to some unknown degree operative (Graham, 1972).

While the superiority of longitudinal data are generally recognized for establishing clear causal links, the role of such data in the study of illness behaviour is particularly crucial. Much confusion and conflicting findings in the field arise from cross-sectional multivariate analyses that ignore the essential dynamic features of the illness experience and coping associated with it.

Take, for example, the issue of denial in illness. Much effort is wasted in attempting to assess whether denial in the case of myocardial infarction, cancer, etc. is a useful defensive reaction. Viewing illness behaviour as a dynamic process, however, reveals that the question is poorly conceptualized and that efforts to answer it are often misguided. Illness experience is part of a continuing process of adaptation in which the individual's efforts to cope are linked in various ways with the particular dimensions of the threat, and both change over time. Thus, at the initial stage of threat following the occurrence of a serious heart attack, where life may be in the balance, denial may effectively serve to reduce distress and to increase the probabilities of survival. Denial at the time of early symptoms, in contrast, may be life-threatening. As patients emerge from the critical period and must face the longer term challenges of their illness and rehabilitation efforts, denial may further restrict access to essential information and needed care. A more refined and realistic approach is to examine how denial functions differently at varying stages of illness, and its consequences as it interacts with other factors.

Much attention is now being devoted to patients' appraisals of their symptoms, the assumptions they make about causes, and how responses to medical advice are conditioned by the 'naïve' theories that patients use to understand their bodily responses. Studies consistently demonstrate major inconsistencies between physicians' expectations and assumptions and patients' responses, resulting in poor communication and difficulties in treatment. Leventhal and colleagues (1980, 1986) find, for example, that while physicians assume that patients with hypertension cannot make judgements of their blood pressure, many patients feel confident in their abilities to assess when their blood pressure is high or low and they adjust their treatment regimens accordingly. Knowing the physician's view, they withhold their assumptions or information about modifications of regimen. Understanding illness theories used by patients thus offers potential for improved communication, more appropriate therapeutic instruction, better treatment regimens, and enhanced adherence to medical advice.

One of the most persistent observations in the epidemiological literature concerns the substantial relationships among reports of physical morbidity, psychological symptoms and self-assessments of health. In one sense, these relationships may be a result of dualism in our language and conceptualizations; there is only a single body but we talk in parallel languages about it (Graham, 1967). At least three central hypotheses have emerged about the relationship between physical and psychological symptoms, each correct to some degree. First, the enormity of serious physical illness causes psychological distress and perhaps also some psychiatric illnesses among vulnerable persons. Secondly, it has been known for decades that major and persistent psychological stress predisposes individuals to physical illness (Dohrenwend & Dohrenwend, 1974, 1981). While there has been active controversy as to whether these effects are specific to a limited set of diagnoses (Graham, 1972) or are relevant to all diagnoses and bodily systems, few seriously doubt that the 'psychosomatic hypothesis' is in some sense valid. The problem consists less in the validity of the insight and more in our incapacities to conceptualize such relationships in a manner promoting increased understanding and improved interventions. A third hypothesis is that certain predispositions of the individual, whether shaped by biology, culture or particular psychological histories, increase the sensitivity or vulnerability of individuals to both physical and psychological symptoms. In our current work we focus on one such predisposition—the tendency to introspect, for example, to be particularly concerned with one's thoughts and feelings. This predisposition is shaped by both culture and social relations, and interacts with varying aspects of social situations.

Determinants of Alternative Expression Patterns

People experience many troubles and tensions that culminate in a variety of adaptations, including physical illness, psychological disorder, and a wide range of attack, escape and risk-taking behaviour. Biology and culture are clearly major limiting factors on how such internal states are expressed. However, a large proportion of what is viewed as illness in modern society appears to be the end point of a process with a variety of alternative pathways. It is estimated that as many as 50% of patients entering medical care have symptoms and complaints that do not fit the International Classification of Diseases, and many others are motivated in seeking care by problems and symptoms other than those with which they present (White, 1970). This suggests the limitations of medical knowledge to some extent, but it also reflects the fact that going to a doctor is part of a process of illness behaviour, involving such factors as felt need, perception, appraisal, definition, attribution of cause, and decision-making.

To the epidemiologist, who begins with a medical definition of a case and not with the processes that lead to its social definition, there are many anomalous findings. Why, for example, are rates of depression, neurotic disturbance, demoralization, and the use of medication relatively high among women, and alcoholism, hard drug use, and violence particularly high among men? Are these independent observations, or is there an underlying process leading to alternative pathways of expression? Why, among populations such as the Chinese, are affective expressions of depression uncommon but the somatic components relatively frequent? Why are rates of suicide among Blacks in the United States relatively low, but rates of homicide so high? An understanding of such questions requires inquiries into culture, social situations and personal predispositions.

A wide range of findings indicates that, in many instances, individuals are unaware of the factors which influence their decisions and actions, even when questioned immediately after the event, and they often deny that such influences affected them even when such influences are identified (Nisbett & Wilson, 1970). Observations of this kind are more comprehensible if we take note of the fact that effective adaptation is often facilitated by the normalization of disruptive or uncomfortable situations and maintenance of the perception of a regular flow of activities. Successful coping often requires the illusion that major changes are limited in impact and that the continuity of the individual persists without major alteration (Mechanic, 1970; Davis, 1963). In contrast to crisis, successful coping involves barely perceptible changes in which the response to challenge becomes part of the ordinary. To be too self-aware of change, and how one is being influenced, is itself stressful (Mechanic, 1962). While people may be altered dramatically over time in dealing with illness or difficult life events, it often serves their interests to perceive that little has changed and to believe that their behaviour arises from acceptable and readily understandable causes. By examining the factors which contribute to distortion, students of illness behaviour enhance their understanding of their subject matter, since distortion is part of the process of defining, struggling with, and coping with potential illness challenges.

Sociocultural Influences

The extraordinary differences among cultures in characterizations of illness, conceptions of causation, and modes of treatment are substantially documented in the anthropological literature (Harwood, 1981). Even in modern populations one finds an interesting blend of sophisticated scientific ideas and folk wisdom learned from close peers and through intuitive processes. Such cultural content affects the recognition and conceptualization of symptoms, the vocabularies for communication, modes and content of expression, and the range of remedial efforts. Even limited historical study reveals how substantially expressions of distress and illness are transformed from one era to another.

The expression of illness through psychological and social vocabularies is a relatively modern phenomenon coexistent with a growth of personal self-awareness and broad self-expression. Female hysteria, for example, characterized by fainting, conversion reactions and 'kicking about' has virtually disappeared in the urban modern environment, although vestiges of the disorder are still seen occasionally in isolated rural cultures that are relatively psychologically unsophisticated and repressive. One interpretation of the disappearance of hysteria is that it no longer brings a sympathetic response from the social environment and is suspect not only among physicians but also among sophisticated persons more generally (Veith, 1970). But, while the dramatic histrionics of hysteria are rarely seen, more mundane expressions of the somatization of distress are ubiquitous and constitute a major load on the medical care system in all nations.

In any historical period the prevailing norms and ideologies encourage or constrain the selection among alternative modes of tension reduction. People facing personal troubles draw on existing sociocultural conceptions of the nature of these troubles and what one might do about them. At any point in time there may be more or less social consensus surrounding the definition of the problem, beliefs about cause, and conceptions of possible remedies. These shape how people view their troubles and what actions they contemplate. Personal tension, for example, may be defined alternatively as resulting from physical illness, personality deficiencies, moral dilemmas, cultural inhibitions, or social exploitation. The availability of reference groups that adhere to particular definitions and provide social support is essential to the maintenance of particular interpretations (Greenley et al. 1976; Kadushin, 1966, 1969). The development of women's consciousness groups in Western nations is a case in point. Prior to such developments, many women experiencing distress and dissatisfaction came to psychiatrists complaining of unhappiness and feelings of inadequacy as wives, mothers and women. The problem was viewed primarily as a unique personal problem resulting from the client's personality and social development. With the growth of the women's movement such feelings are increasingly seen as a consequence of constraining role expectations, exploitative role relationships and blocked opportunities to achieve aspirations, and it is not difficult to find many women reinforcing this conception and providing social support. Thus personal distress is increasingly being redefined as a commonly shared social problem. Similar redefinitions are increasingly applied by the aged, the handicapped and homosexuals. This is not to suggest that such groups do not have serious personal problems or handicaps. But such examples demonstrate that the construction of health and disease is a social process, often arbitrary in conceptualization (Dubos, 1959).

The Social Situation

Illness behaviour arises in response to circumstances that challenge the ongoing homeostasis. People are extraordinarily adaptive, but some changes in the situation, whether arising within the organism or from external factors, induce self-consciousness and appraisal, and require assessments about the nature of the problem, its causes and the strategies to be initiated. These responses are both cognitive and affective, concerned with understanding the changes and maintaining emotional equilibrium.

Illness behaviour is more than a psychological response among persons faced with a situation calling for assessment. It also arises in response to troubling social situations and may serve as an effective means of achieving release from social expectations, as an excuse for failure, or as a way of obtaining a variety of privileges including monetary compensation. Moreover, the physician and other health personnel may be an important source of social support and may be particularly important for patients lacking strong social ties. A vague complaint of illness may be one way of seeking reassurance and support through a recognized and socially acceptable relationship when it is difficult for the patient to confront the underlying problem in an unambiguous way without displaying weaknesses and vulnerabilities contrary to expected and learned behaviour patterns. Balint (1957) and others have noted that the presenting symptoms may be of no special importance, but serve to establish the relationship between the patient and the doctor.

A vast number of doctor-patient contacts involve symptoms and illnesses that are widely distributed in the population and that are more frequently untreated than treated (White et al. 1961). Thus the decision to seek care is frequently a result of contingencies surrounding the perception of symptoms. Perceptions of oneself as ill and seeking care may provide self-justification when potential failure poses much greater symbolic threats to the individual's self-esteem than the process of being ill or dependent (Cole & Lejeune, 1972).

A related issue is the difficulty experienced by some patients of differentiating symptoms of psychological origin from symptoms of particular diseases. Many illnesses, or effects of medications prescribed for dealing with them, produce feelings comparable with those associated with stress and psychopathology. Such symptoms as fatigue, restlessness and poor appetite, for example, may result either from depression or from an acute infectious disease. When both occur concurrently, patients may attribute the effects of one to another. There is an indication, for example, that long convalescence from acute infectious disease may result from the attribution of symptoms caused by depression to the acute condition (Imboden et al. 1961). This complicates not only the patient's recovery but also the physician's perception and management of the patient.

Personal Predispositions

The variability in patient behaviour in a given subculture, despite the similarity of symptoms, also reflects major differences in psychological orientations and predispositions. At a simple level, people vary in their tolerance for discomfort, in the knowledge, information and understanding which they have about the illness process, and in the specific ways in which bodily indications affect needs and ongoing social roles. People seem to vary a great deal in their subjective response to pain and discomfort, although there appears to be much less difference in physical thresholds. Much research has demonstrated that pain has an important subjective component, and there is no clear relationship between the amount of tissue damage and the degree of discomfort reported by the patient (Beecher, 1959; Melzack, 1973). What people know, believe, and think about illness, of course, affects what symptoms they think are important, what is viewed as more or less serious, and what one should do.

We are engaged at present in research on one specific predisposition—introspectiveness (a tendency to think about oneself, and one's motivations and feelings)—which we believe is fundamental to understanding appraisal and illness behaviour (Mechanic, 1983). Over the years there have been numerous efforts to measure personal traits which characterize individuals who display an exaggerated illness dependency. During the height of dominance of psychodynamic ideas in psychiatry such individuals were commonly characterized as 'neurotic' and, more recently, as 'worried wells', but neither concept provides an adequate conceptualization of such personal traits or the processes by which exaggerated illness patterns develop.

The concept of enduring personal traits has increasingly been called into question. There was little evidence that personal characteristics were stable across situations or over time. While the difficulty of demonstrating stability may, in part, be methodological (Epstein, 1979), current data suggest that it is more appropriate to speak of predispositions or orientations which may be operative only under certain conditions.

Introspection appears to be an important orientation in the illness behaviour process. Results from research programmes investigating such varied issues as self-esteem, objective self-awareness, pain response, behaviour and health, private self-consciousness and ego defense processes all support the hypothesis that attention to self increases the prevalence of reported psychological and physical symptoms and negative self-evaluations (Mechanic, 1983).

I first made this observation more than 20 years ago, but did not fully appreciate its significance. We had asked mothers of young children to keep detailed illness diaries for themselves and other family members, requiring responses to a specific symptom inventory each day. We had some difficulty in gaining cooperation and, when we questioned mothers who were reluctant, some indicated that the attention to symptoms required by completing the diary, made them feel worse. What was so evident phenomenologically to the individuals involved has now been clearly established in a variety of laboratory studies under controlled conditions.

In a variety of studies examining introspection we find that individuals with such an orientation report more physical and psychological distress, are more upset by stressful life events, and use more medical, psychiatric and other helping services (Mechanic, 1979, 1980; Greenley & Mechanic, 1976; Mechanic & Hansell, 1983). This orientation, we believe, is conditioned by sociocultural factors and childhood socialization, and it may be triggered by particular situational events (Mechanic, 1972). More recently, we have found that individuals with an introspective orientation are more reactive to interpersonal adversities affecting significant others, while those less directed to their internal states show less distress (Mechanic & Hansell, 1983).

The fact that people cope much of the time without awareness is a central point in understanding personal and social adaptation. To become aware, to become self-conscious, is an indication of more than a routine problem, a greater challenge, a break in the flow of normal activity. People can at any time be confronted with serious illness or personal tragedy. But it is not psychologically economical to worry about what one cannot predict or control, and individuals maintain a sense of invulnerability by inattention to potential threat (Janis, 1951; Mechanic, 1972). Too much inattention or denial distracts attention from essential information acquisition and planning, but we maintain our comfort by a considerable filtering of potentially threatening information.

Individuals who are more introspective probably know themselves better, and perhaps have a better understanding of the influences that affect them, but they also appear more uncomfortable with themselves and their life situations.They are more prone to react to threatening situations and more likely to define many common, self-limited bodily sensations as symptoms. While introspectiveness, properly guided, may be associated with valued consequences—such as creativity, sensitivity, and empathy with others, and artistic expression—it also appears to exaggerate the experience of distress and illness.

Introspectiveness is only one of many personal inclinations or traits that may interact with perceptions of threat, coping and the illness experience. Such traits may profoundly affect perceptions and response, the course of the illness experience, and the quality of adaptation. They also may affect the propensity to view oneself as ill, the degree of personal suffering experienced, and the degree to which common bodily signals are conceptualized in a threatening way.

In sum, illness behaviour involves a complex interaction between the quality of bodily dysfunction, the sociocultural and psychological orientations brought by individuals to their situation, and the unique demands of the immediate social context. Epidemiological studies show that most people can elicit symptoms comparable with those most commonly presented in medical interactions. The challenge is to gain a better understanding of the question posed so clearly by Michael Balint in helping general practitioners to understand their patients' behaviour. Why has the patient chosen to emphasize this time, and this set of symptoms? The fact that similar, and even more serious, symptoms were evident on other occasions when no comparable behaviour took place remains the core of the puzzle we strive to understand.

References

Balint, M. (1957). *The Doctor, His Patient and the Illness*. International Universities Press: New York.

Beecher, H. K. (1959). *Measurement of Subjective Responses: Quantitative Effects of Drugs*. Oxford University Press: New York.

Cole, S. & Lejeune, R. (1972). Illness and the legitimation of failure. *American Sociological Review* 37, 347–356.

Davis, F. (1963). *Passage Through Crisis: Polio Victims and Their Families*. Bobbs-Merrill Co.: Indianapolis.

Dohrenwend, B. S. & Dohrenwend, B. P. (eds.) (1974). *Stressful Life Events: Their Nature and Effects*. Wiley Interscience: New York.

Dohrenwend, B. S. & Dohrenwend, B. P. (eds.) (1981). *Stressful Life Events and Their Contexts*. Rutgers University Press: New Brunswick, NJ.

Dubos, R. (1959). *Mirage of Health, Utopias, Progress and Biological Change*. Harper and Bros: New York.

Epstein, S. (1979). The stability of behavior. I: On predicting most of the people much of the time. *Journal of Personality and Social Psychiatry* 37, 1097–1126.

Graham, D. T. (1967). Health, disease, and the mind-body problem. linguistic parallelism. *Psychosomatic Medicine* 29, 52–71.

Graham, D. T. (1972). Psychosomatic medicine. In *Handbook of Psychophysiology* (ed. N. S. Greenfield and R. A. Sternbach). pp. 839–924. Holt, Rinehart and Winston: New York.

Greenley, J. R. & Mechanic, D. (1976). Social selection in seeking help for psychological problems. *Journal of Health and Social Behaviour* 17, 249–262.

Harwood, A. (ed.) (1981). *Ethnicity and Medical Care*. Harvard University Press: Cambridge, Mass.

Imboden, J. B., Canter, A. & Cluff, L. (1961). Symptomatic recovery from medical disorders. *Journal of the American Medical Association* 178, 1182–1184.

Janis, I. L. (1951). *Air War and Emotional Stress: Psychological Studies of Bombing and Civilian Defense*. McGraw-Hill: New York.

Kadushin, C. (1966). The friends and supporters of psychotherapy: on social circles in urban life. *American Sociological Review* 31, 786–802.

Kadushin, C. (1969). *Why People Go to Psychiatrists*. Atherton: New York.

Leventhal, H., Meyer, D. & Nerenz, D. (1980). The common-sense representation of illness danger. In *Medical Psychology*, Vol. 2 (ed. D. Rachman), pp. 7–30. Pergamon: New York.

Leventhal, H., Prohaska, T. H. & Hirschman, R. S. (1986). Preventive health behavior across the life-span. In *Preventing Health Risk Behaviors and Promoting Coping with Illness (1985)*, Vol. 8 (ed. J. C. Rosen and L. J. Solomon). University of New England: Hanover, N.H.

Mechanic, D. (1962). *Students Under Stress: A Study in the Social Psychology of Adaptation*. Free Press: New York. (Republished by the University of Wisconsin Press with a new introduction, 1978.)

Mechanic, D. (1970). Some problems in developing a social psychology of adaptation to stress. In *Social and Psychological Factors in Stress* (ed. J. E. McGrath), pp. 104–123. Holt, Rinehart and Winston: New York.

Mechanic, D. (1972). Social psychologic factors affecting the presentation of bodily complaints. *New England Journal of Medicine* 286, 1132–1139.

Mechanic, D. (1978). *Medical Sociology* (second edn.) Free Press: New York.

Mechanic, D. (1979). Development of psychological distress among young adults. *Archives of General Psychiatry* 36, 1233–1239.

Mechanic, D. (1980). The experience and reporting of common physical complaints. *Journal of Health and Social Behaviour* 21, 146–155.

Mechanic, D. (1983). Adolescent health and illness behaviour: hypotheses for the study of distress in youth. *Journal of Human Stress* 9, 4–13.

Mechanic, D. & Hansell, S. (1983). Adolescent introspectiveness, psychological distress, and physical symptoms. Presented at the 78th Annual Meeting of the American Sociological Association. Detroit, September.

Melzack, R. (1973). *The Puzzle of Pain: Revolution in Theory and Treatment*. Basic Books: New York.

Nisbett, R. N. & Wilson, T. D. (1970). Telling more than we can know: verbal reports of mental processes. *Psychological Review* 84, 231–259.

Veith, I. (1970). *Hysteria: The History of a Disease*. University of Chicago Press: Chicago.

White, K. L. (1970). Evaluation of medical education and health care. In *Community Medicine: Teaching, Research, and Health Care* (ed. W. Lathem and A. Newbery), pp. 241–270. Appleton-Century Crofts: New York.

White, K. L., Williams, T. F. & Greenberg, B. G. (1961). The ecology of medical care. *New England Journal of Medicine* 265, 885–892.

5

Health and Behavior:
Perspectives on Risk Prevention

It is commonly recognized that the vast resources our nation invests in health care come too late in most instances to do more than ameliorate the course of disease and disability. Much energy and money are spent on halfway technologies that save and extend lives but involve large economic, social, and psychological costs for the community, the patient, and the family. Prevention is, of course, a better strategy in every sense, but if it is to be more than an empty slogan, it must be built on a strong infrastructure of basic research in the biological and behavioral sciences that directs intervention in meaningful ways.

Those working in the curative health arena not uncommonly express impatience with the advocates of prevention. In their view, there is not much we know how to prevent beyond current efforts. In most circumstances involving death and disability—as in the case of heart disease, cancer, and mental disorder—basic scientific knowledge of etiology is inadequate and interventions remain problematic. Where identifiable risk factors can be controlled, the barriers in doing so often relate to the difficulty of altering cultural patterns and individual behavior, and on resolving conflicts with important social, economic, and political agendas. While there is much we can still do in smoking and hypertension control, immunization, prenatal and child care efforts, and other selected areas where interventions can make a difference, the barriers typically are not in our knowledge but rather in our politics. It is unlikely that we would ignore any technical intervention that prevented or clearly limited disease. The gap is mainly in how we respond to indirect evidence of risk factors, particularly when such responses involve economic or political costs for powerful interest groups.

The recognition that patterns of disease and mortality substantially

70

depend on our environment and social structure is now commonplace. While medicine has brought many achievements, and has contributed immeasurably to disease management and a sense of personal security, it contributes within narrow constraints set by economic and cultural patterns, values, and the general state of technology. Despite these constraints, progress in promoting health has been impressive. In this century longevity has increased substantially in all developed countries and in many underdeveloped ones, in large part due to improved food production, standards of nutrition, and economic circumstances. In the first half of the century, progress was most notable in the control of infectious disease and infant death, but in many countries dramatic changes occurred as well in chances of survival at older ages. In the United States, life expectancy remained relatively constant after 1955 for a number of years, but in more recent years considerable gains have been achieved in expected survival throughout the life span. Age-specific mortality for most causes, including cardiovascular disease, has decreased reflecting a wide range of factors associated with standards of living, medical progress, and changes in behavior. The precise contributors remain unclear.

A Framework for Understanding Risk Factors and Prevention

Much of our understanding of risk factors derives from epidemiological studies that provide leads for more focused investigations and experimental and clinical research. Ultimately, the value of an intervention must be assessed through controlled investigations, preferably using random assignment. But even a favorable result in a randomized controlled trial, while enhancing prevention, does not establish understanding. Knowledge of disease processes is firm when we understand basic processes and can demonstrate such understanding experimentally.

Epidemiology views disease and disorder through time and space, working against the parochialism of short-term study of selected, and frequently biased, samples. The approach makes clear the necessity to differentiate factors contributing initially to illness (incidence) from those that affect the course of disorder (prevalence). Moreover, it facilitates differentiation between the character of disorders and processes of seeking and utilizing help. Thus it is a useful way of examining etiological factors, those factors that affect prognosis, and the processes of acquiring medical and other types of care.

In preventing disease, ideally we want to proceed on the basis of specific understanding of disease mechanisms, but indirect evidence is often useful. In the classic cases of Snow's investigation of cholera and Goldberger's study of pellagra, it was possible to prevent the occurrence of disease through water control and dietary measures, respectively, despite the fact that the specific agents remained unidentified. More contemporary examples include smoking, weight control, diet, and exercise. But these examples illustrate the weaknesses as well as the utility of indirect knowledge. Advice on dietary precautions has changed over time, is inconsistent from one disease to another, and in the aggregate is often confusing. The advantages of precise knowledge in targeting more effective interventions should be clear.

In examining trends in morbidity and longevity, general characteristics of populations are often better predictors than biological or psychological markers other than sex and age. The frequency of disease and mortality increases over the life span, and women retain an advantage in longevity of approximately eight years. A remarkable number of studies also show disease and mortality linked with schooling, poverty, marital status, social and community integration, employment availability, and stable living conditions. The measures vary from one study to another, controls are often absent or inadequate, and cause and effect confused or unclear; but the consistency of results across populations, theoretical perspectives, methods, and measures suggest that these indirect associations are worthy of our attention.

Schooling, one of the best predictors of good health, longevity, and use of preventive and other health services, is an instructive example. Schooling is substantially correlated with income, but invariably has effects on health beyond income. Education is associated with life chances and many other attributes associated with health, including habits, coping capacities, and self-esteem. While it is plausible that intervening variables would explain the education effects, no study yet has been successful in doing so. It has been suggested that perhaps the most effective way of promoting health is to increase levels of education and income, but the costs and inefficiencies are high and political barriers are considerable, relative to identifying specific influential causative factors.

One of the most neglected, but important, predictors of health is marital status, comparable in effect to that of a person's sex. While marriage favors men more than women, both gain appreciably relative to the unmarried, particularly relative to divorced persons. Some of the outcomes result from the alienation and distress accompanying divorce, exemplified by excessive drinking, accidents, and violence. But the marriage effect is nonspecific, affecting disease rates and mortality more extensively. Marriage, of course, is a powerful social institution, and it not only typically provides established routines in respect to nutrition, sleep, and other matters, but also involves strong expectations, personal commitments, and goals beyond one's own interests.

The marital status variable is a complex one and illustrates the risks of focusing on broad associations in contrast to specific etiologic agents. Marital status and marital stability involve strong social selection factors, and the meaning of marriage changes in varying age cohorts with historical shifts. It would seem premature to argue that maintaining marriage is a positive goal for health maintenance, but such claims are made by even relatively sophisticated advocates (Lynch, 1977). This advocacy is not unlike that for changing behavior types (Friedman & Rosenman, 1974), an uncertain endeavor deriving from the growing literature linking Type A behavior pattern to coronary heart disease.

Findings in respect to religious participation, psychological well-being, and social integration all probably share a common core. There is no particular reason why persons attending church should live longer than those who do not, although churchgoing is probably related to greater conventionality and thus more regularity in lifestyles. Moreover, religious participation may be associated with positive health behavior in respect to smoking, drinking, and other risks, consequences clearly apparent among Mormons, Seventh Day Adventists, and other religious groups. Religious participation also implies a commitment, a sense of belonging, and a network of social relationships many studies show to be important in dealing with adversities and in maintaining health. Recent sophisticated studies demonstrate that intimacy and social networks not only protect against the occurrence of depression (Brown & Harris, 1978) and other morbid conditions, but also promote longevity (House, Robbins, & Metzner, 1982).

Integration into larger social networks of associations not only provides an arena for personal and social commitment, but also may offer an established and health-promoting routine, social support, and tangible assistance when needed. Group association may serve as a basis for personal gratification and self-esteem as well. While the concept of social integration implies a variety of causal interpretations, studies more specifically focused on psychological distress demonstrate clearly that personal distress is always associated with a range of bodily symptoms.

Poor health and mortality also are associated with involuntary disruptions in people's adaptations to their environment, including such events as unemployment, forced retirement, and involuntary relocations. Employment, of course, is related to economic as well as psychological factors, but for many—if not a majority of—people, work provides a sense of meaning, participation, and involvement with others central to one's life. The causal sequence is complex, since unemployment or retirement may be accompanied by a significant reduction in income and a change in lifestyle, and aging, which brings more health problems, need to be taken into account. Retirement as defined in our society, by itself, does not appear to be a risk factor if aging effects and prior health status are controlled (Ekerdt, Baden, Bossé, & Dibbs, 1983).

The significance of "meaning" affecting biological events is illustrated in an intriguing study of "death dips" prior to events of important cultural significance (Phillips & Feldman, 1973). A "death dip" is the occurrence of fewer deaths than expected. Studies of various groups of famous people show that they are more likely to die following a birthday than before, and the more famous the individuals, the larger the death dip. Birthdays of famous people are more likely to be publicly celebrated, or to be associated with tokens of respect and admiration. A death dip prior to presidential elections, and for Jewish populations prior to the Jewish Day of Atonement, have also been demonstrated. Although the biological mechanism remains unclear, people can postpone their deaths, an observation commonly made by clinicians working with critically ill patients. That death can be very much accelerated through psychological processes has long been recognized, dating back to Walter Cannon's discussion of voodoo death.

Finally, there are abundant historical data tracing patterns of disease and mortality following forced relocations of populations, the movement of populations from rural to urban living, and the movement of elderly patients from one institution to another. While these data tend to be sketchy, they depict populations experiencing disorientation with rapid social change in their surroundings. Such periods appear to be characterized by high rates of disease and mortality until the population adjusts to its new surroundings. Elderly persons moved from one institution to another die beyond usual expectations, as do persons losing a spouse. John Cassel, an eminent epidemiologist who devoted many years to such questions (Cassel, 1970), suggested that rapid social change has undermined the adaptive capacities of populations that have evolved over long periods of time, and the effects of changes such as movement from rural to urban factory life have been evident even for the offspring of those initially affected (Cassel & Tyroler, 1961).

At a more manageable level for rigorous research, there has evolved a vast body of evidence linking life change events with the occurrence of illness (Dohrenwend & Dohrenwend, 1974, 1981). An important underlying hypothesis is that major changes require adjustments that strain the biological system and result in adverse health outcomes. While the debate continues on the types of events that most dramatically affect health and the causal processes involved, the literature supports the assumption that major discontinuity in living conditions increases vulnerability to ill health.

Examining Intervening Processes: Some Examples

The types of broad relationships I have described only take us partway in identifying risk factors that can be efficiently modified. Much of the challenge remains in identifying intervening processes and how biological propensities interact with personal traits and sociocultural and situational influences. Here I turn to some of our own efforts to understand personal appraisals of health status, factors encouraging sensitivity to symptoms and psychological distress, and determinants of health behavior.

In 1961, I selected a sample of mother-child pairs from the population of Madison, Wisconsin, and independent data were obtained from mothers, children, teachers, and official school records. In addition, 198 mothers completed daily illness diaries for themselves and their children for 15 days following their interviews. The sample included all fourth-grade children in five schools and half of the eighth-grade students, chosen randomly, from the three middle schools in the city. The socio-economic distributions of the fourth- and eighth-grade populations were substantially the same. The sample of 350 mother-child pairs constituted 93% of the eligible sample population. Mothers were interviewed at home, whereas information from the children was obtained in school (Mechanic, 1964).

The 1961 study provided a variety of interesting findings (Mechanic, 1964, 1968; Mechanic & Newton, 1965). Perhaps most impressive was the difficulty in demonstrating the transmission of the content of health behavior from mother to child. Whereas we found many such relationships, the amount of variance accounted for was small and the pattern of results was not fully consistent. The best predictors of the children's illness behaviors were age and sex. As in other studies, we found that mothers' reports about themselves and their children were often correlated; mothers under stress, for example, reported not only more symptoms for themselves but also for their children, and they were more likely to phone the doctor concerning their children's health. However, there were fewer and smaller associations when data were independently obtained from mothers, children, teachers, and official records, subsequently found to be true in many areas of study. These initial findings alerted us to the importance of respondent effects, particularly when people report not only for themselves but also for others, and in our subsequent studies of medical care we have tried to obtain data for independent and dependent variables from separate sources. In 1977, we located 333 of the original 350 children (95%). Of the remaining 17, 6 had died and 11 could not be found. Of those located, 302 (91%) completed detailed questionnaires.

Neither our data nor other studies find much support for the view that various types of health behavior reflect an underlying dimension of responsibility for health maintenance. However, one approach to the study of positive health behavior is to score respondents on the extent to which they adhere to behavior believed to be consistent with health status (Belloc & Breslow, 1972). Thus, we constructed an index based on eight measures of health response, including smoking, drinking, seat belt use, exercise, physical activity, risk taking, preventive medical behavior, and preparation for emergencies (Mechanic & Cleary, 1980). Men had lower scores on this index, reflecting more drinking and risk taking, and less preventive medical behavior. Other predictors of high scores on positive health behavior included education, concern with health, and a conventional behavioral orientation. Perhaps most interesting was the fact that both psychological well-being and subjective assessments of excellent physical health were associated with high scores on positive health behavior. Whereas a selection hypothesis is plausible in that physical stamina may be associated with exercise and physical activity, it is more difficult to explain why poorer subjective health status should result in smoking, failure to use seat belts, or less preventive medical care.

Our analyses lead us to speculate that patterns of health behavior tend to be part of lifestyles related to the ability to anticipate problems, to mobilize to meet them, and to cope actively. A measure of psychological distress (symptoms indicating anxiety and depression), for example, is significantly related to five components of the behavior index: drinking (.21); smoking (.25); failure to use seat belts (.16); lower physical activity ($-.23$); and less exercise ($-.23$). Behaviors like smoking and drinking may, in part, be efforts to alleviate distress, whereas others, like physical inactivity and failure to use seat belts, may reflect poor anticipation and inertia. Persons with poorer health behavior also appear to be less integrated into the conventional culture.

These data are consistent with the more global description I presented earlier. The significance is not, as some believe, that there is an easily modifiable, underlying trait of responsibility for health. More important, I think, the data emphasize the extent to which behavior derives from an overall living pattern, reflecting social values, psychological well-being, and integration into a dominant cultural mode. To the extent to which there is a personal orientation to good health practices, all evidence to date suggests that this orientation is at best loosely organized, with each particular behavior sequence having relatively unique determinants. Different health behaviors are not only usually modestly correlated but are, in some instances, negatively associated. Persons, for example, who are physically active—a commendable goal for encouraging positive health— also take more risks involving danger.

Vulnerability to Psychological and Physical Distress

We have been engaged for many years in studies of illness behavior and the individual's use of medical and psychiatric services. These studies, and the literature more generally, indicate that a relatively limited proportion of the population makes a large and disproportionate demand for services, and that such patients constitute not only the very ill in a medical sense but also many who complain of physical and psychological distress but have no demonstrable clinical illness. Our follow-up study of children allowed us to examine such states of distress in a developmental context.

We used two measures of distress: the first, an index of psychological distress with seven items depicting anxiety and depression; the second, a summary measure of 15 common physical complaints. These two measures are correlated .42, and neither is associated with sex in this sample. Since the results are similar for the two dependent variables, I focus on psychological distress, but will later briefly note some differences in determinants of the two types of complaints.

These dependent variables, typical of measures used in psychiatric epidemiology, do not measure illness as such, but there is considerable disagreement as to what they actually represent. It has been suggested that they reflect demoralization, self-dissatisfaction, or a quasi-neurosis, and may either accompany or be independent of tangible illness. High scores on these measures appear to tap the diffuse neuroses that have been of particular interest to psychodynamically oriented ego psychologists and psychiatrists. The index used in our study had an average correlation of .56 with five other variables denoting low psychological well-being: self-description of unhappiness (.46), description of low spirits (−.44), degree of worry about eight specified life problems (.56), high neuroticism on the Eysenck scale (.77), and low self-esteem (−.59). Our index was also correlated .41 with respondents' reports in 1977 that they had emotional problems, nervous trouble, or chronic "nerves."

The theoretical hypothesis used in the analysis was that the sense of distress measured by our index was shaped by three aspects: (1) body sensations, symptoms, or feelings different from those ordinarily experienced; (2) social stress; and (3) cognitions appraising what a person is feeling (Mechanic, 1972). Changes in body sensations, I argue, increase self-awareness, and stress contributes to body arousal and psychological disorientation further motivating attention to inner feelings. The regression analyses are consistent with the conclusion that factors focusing the child's attention on internal states and teaching a pattern of internal monitoring contribute to a distress syndrome. Respondents with such syndromes were more likely to come from families in which the mother was more upset and symptomatic, the child had more common physical symptoms such as colds and sore throats, and attention was directed to such symptoms by keeping the child home from school. Moreover, the data do not support the hypothesis that adulthood distress syndromes are simply a continuous pattern of illness from childhood to young adulthood. Although learned internal monitoring appears to be an important aspect of distress, it is only a vulnerability factor. The regression model based on the four most influential 1961 predictors of distress, childhood physical symptoms, school absence, and two maternal measures, explains only 9% of the variance. Whether a distress syndrome will develop depends on many additional influences, such as the degree of psychological and bodily dysfunction, adverse life experience, and influences that reinforce a focus on internal feeling states.

There is increasing experimental evidence that simply drawing a subject's attention to some aspect of bodily functioning results in an increased prevalence of symptom reporting (Pennebaker & Skelton, 1978), and experimentally induced self-awareness most commonly results in negative evaluation (Wicklund, 1975). Thus, it is plausible that persons who focus on feelings and bodily changes will be more likely to experience disturbing states. In an earlier epidemiological study of Wisconsin students, Greenley and Mechanic (1976) found that respondents high on a scale of identification with introspective others not only reported more psychological symptoms, but also were more likely to use medical, counseling, and other formal helping services. In the child follow-up study, introspectiveness was measured by a scale in which respondents indicated the degree to which they were "sensitive and introspective," "worried about meaning in life," and were "interested in psychology." Scores on this scale are correlated .47 with the distress measure despite the fact that the items do not directly measure symptoms and describe everyday concerns. The effect is approximately the same for each item in the scale. When added to various regression models of distress, introspectiveness retains its strength as a predictor, overshadowing all other predictors.

As one might anticipate, the introspectiveness score is related to parental variables similar to those predicting adult distress, particularly measures of parental negative behavior toward the child. Conceivably, such a pattern of concern with self and self-scrutiny results when familial patterns are disrupted, and such self-appraisal usually culminates in negative self-evaluation.

As noted earlier, our scales of psychological distress and of reporting common physical symptoms are substantially correlated, have many similar predictors, and are amenable to a common theoretical interpretation. Two possible important determinants that differentiate persons who favor psychological and those who favor physical complaining are actual adult experience with symptoms and illness on the one hand, and cultural influences on the definition of illness on the other. Whereas reporting physical symptoms is culturally more neutral, reporting psychological symptoms is more dependent on social acceptability. Social desirability response bias was significantly associated with reporting psychological symptoms (−.18), but was not significantly associated with reporting physical symptoms (−.06). In contrast, reports of chronic illness, bed disability days, and tendency to get sick were more highly correlated with physical symptoms than with psychological reports. We believe that the types of perceptual and definitional processes that have been described filter objective physical experience and cultural influences.

Reinforcing Factors

I have concentrated thus far on internal factors that either reinforce or distract attention from bodily concerns, but external reinforcements are equally important. The literature on behavior change attests to the ease of achieving short-term modifications of behavior, but rarely do these effects persist for long periods with significant proportions of the population. Evidently frequent and repeated external reinforcement is an essential aspect of desired behavioral continuity (Haggerty, 1977). Such reinforcement may come through family settings, peer relations, the work place, and a variety of other life contexts—a fact generally appreciated. It is less commonplace to understand the extent to which effective reinforcements, or their obverse, are implicit in the social and cultural systems we take for granted, and they may be far more powerful, in part, because they are not intended to bring about behavior consistent with a public agenda. Good health practices that occur not because they are good for health, but because they are consistent with how people choose to live, are more significant than any efforts we can reasonably make to change behavior. Promoting health is, thus, in large part an effort in social and cultural change and, most fundamentally, involves the conscious and unconscious designs for living that people follow. These conclusions in no way denigrate the importance of smoking control, treatment of obesity, or whatever; but they alert us to the limitations of our own efforts. We can anticipate major difficulties in preventive efforts if we fail to take account of the degree to which behaviors we wish to promote or change are embedded in routine habits and social patterns. The most powerful facilitation of positive health behavior is to integrate successfully desired patterns with the culture of natural supportive groups. Behaviors routinely reinforced by the social context are more robust than those requiring special programs.

In many instances the promotion of health is more likely to be successful through technological or regulatory means than through behavior change. If we wish to reduce accidents and deaths among teenagers—an extremely high-risk group for auto deaths—we do better by delaying the legal age for driving than by driver's education (Robertson, 1983). Even the most elaborate campaigns for seat belt use achieve only modest use. Automatic safety devices and environmental controls frequently offer greater benefits at less cost. In practice, we typically end up with some mix of education, technology, and regulation. Whatever the issue, an aggregate strategy calling upon a number of methods simultaneously offers the best possibilities, particularly when the noxious behavior is personally and socially rewarding in some way. Clearly, we also do better to prevent noxious behaviors initially. Targeting high-risk groups is a sensible priority.

While it is commonplace to give lip service to the role people have in their own health and the importance of health promotion, efforts to understand the causal process affecting these behaviors or to evaluate the impact of varying strategies in preventing or changing such patterns still receive little public support. A model of health promotion based on sound principles of intervention offers as much potential for health maintenance as any curative medical technology. Ironically, there is very little relationship between publicly stated aspirations and rhetoric, and the willingness to finance development of the necessary knowledge and programming for future efforts.

References

Belloc, N. B., & Breslow, L. Relationship of physical health status and health practice. *Preventive Medicine,* 1972, 1, 409–421.

Brown, G. W., & Harris, T. *Social origins of depression: A study of psychiatric disorder in women.* New York: The Free Press, 1978.

Cassel, J. Physical illness in response to stress. In S. Levine and N. A. Scotch (Eds.), *Social stress.* Chicago: Aldine, 1970, pp. 189–209.

Cassel, J., & Tyroler, H. A. Epidemiological studies of social change: Health status and recency of industrialization. *Archives of Environmental Health,* 1961, 3, 25–33.

Dohrenwend, B. S., & Dohrenwend, B. P. (Eds.). *Stressful life events.* New York: John Wiley & Sons, 1974.

Dohrenwend, B. S., & Dohrenwend, B. P. *Stressful life events and their contexts.* New Brunswick, N.J.: Rutgers University Press, 1981.

Ekerdt, D. J, Baden, L., Bossé, R., & Dibbs, E. The effect of retirement on physical health. *American Journal of Public Health,* 1983, 73, 779–783.

Friedman, M. & Rosenman, R. H. *Type A behavior and your heart.* New York: Knopf, 1974.

Greenley, J. R., & Mechanic, D. Social selection in seeking help for psychological problems. *Journal of Health and Social Behavior,* 1976, 17, 249–262.

Haggerty, R. J. Changing life styles to improve health. *Preventive Medicine,* 1977, 6, 276–289.

House, J., Robbins, C., & Metzner, H. L. The association of social relationship and activities with mortality: Prospective evidence from the Tecumseh community health study. *American Journal of Epidemiology,* 1982, 116, 123–140.

Lynch, J. J. *The broken heart: The medical consequences of loneliness.* New York: Basic Books, 1977.

Mechanic, D. The influence of mothers on their children's health attitudes and behavior. *Pediatrics,* 1964, 33, 444–453.

Mechanic, D. *Medical sociology: A selective view.* New York: The Free Press, 1968.

Mechanic, D. Social psychologic factors affecting the presentation of bodily complaints. *New England Journal of Medicine,* 1972, 286, 1132–1139.

Mechanic, D., & Cleary, P. Factors associated with the maintenance of positive health behavior. *Preventive Medicine,* 1980, 9, 805–814.

Mechanic, D., & Newton, M. Some problems in the analysis of morbidity data. *Journal of Chronic Disease,* 1965, 18, 569–580.

Pennebaker, J. W., & Skelton, J. A. Psychological parameters of physical symptoms. *Personality and Social Psychology Bulletin,* 1978, 4, 524–530.

Phillips, D., & Feldman, K. A dip in deaths before ceremonial occasions: Some new relationships between social integration and mortality. *American Sociological Review,* 1973, 38, 678–696.

Robertson, L. S. Injury epidemiology and the reduction of harm. In D. Mechanic (Ed.), *Handbook of health, health care, and the health professions.* New York: The Free Press, 1983.

Wicklund, R. Objective self-awareness. In L. Berkowitz (Ed.), *Advances in experimental social psychology* (Vol. 8). New York: Academic Press, 1975, pp. 233–275.

6

Social Structure and Personal Adaptation: Some Neglected Dimensions

The study of social adaptation is most typically pursued without seriously considering the pervasive influence of social structural variables on personal and social adaptation. Traditional approaches to adaptation have developed from psychodynamic studies and ego psychology, and there has been a continuing tendency to see mastery of the environment in terms of intrapsychic mechanisms that allow individuals to control psychologically the environmental stimuli impinging upon them and to maintain a state of personal comfort. More recently, with growing emphasis on environmental mastery and effective performance, some investigators have broadened their scope of study to include such concerns as the learning and use of skills and the direct manipulation of the environment, but this new development has not been very systematically developed. Almost all stress investigators, irrespective of their orientations, neglect consideration of the relationship between social structure and mastery.

From a social psychological point of view, it has increasingly become apparent to investigators of stress that adaptation must be considered in terms of the relationship between external physical and social demands on the person and his resources to deal with these (McGrath 1970). It has become commonplace to consider the potentialities for adaptation in terms of the fit between person and environment, and even therapeutic approaches are frequently based on achieving a more congruent fit. Because the approach to adaptation has been primarily a psychological one, the person-environment fit usually considered is an attitudinal fit, or one based on how the person perceives himself in relation to the environment. Only more recently has there been greater emphasis on the issue of whether the person's actual skills are capable of dealing with true external demands.

Successful personal adaptation has at least three components at the

82

individual level. First, the person must have the capabilities and skills to deal with the social and environmental demands to which he is exposed; for the sake of simplicity I shall designate these skills as coping capabilities. Such capacities involve the ability not only to react to environmental demands, but also to influence and control the demands to which one will be exposed and at what pace. Second, individuals must be motivated to meet the demands that become evident in their environment. Individuals can escape anxiety and discomfort by lowering their motivation and aspirations, but as we will see later there are many social constraints against this mode of reducing stress. As motivation increases, the consequences of failing to achieve mastery also increase, and level of motivation is frequently an important prerequisite for experiencing psychological discomfort. Third, individuals must have the capabilities to maintain a state of psychological equilibrium so that they can direct their energies and skills to meeting external, in contrast to internal, needs. It should be apparent that much of the psychological literature on adaptation concerns itself with this third dimension—one which I refer to as defense. Although psychologists who have studied stress have viewed defense as an end in itself, it is more reasonable to see defense as a set of mechanisms that facilitates continuing performance and mastery. Defenses that may be very successful in diminishing pain and discomfort may be catastrophic for personal adaptation if they retard the enactment of behavior directed toward real threats in the environment. To put the matter bluntly, such defenses as denial—a persistent and powerful psychological response—will do a drowning man no good!

There is still another kind of person-environment fit that is rarely discussed in the literature on stress and adaptation, but it is probably the most important of all. This fit between the social structure and environmental demands is probably the major determinant of successful social adaptation. Man's abilities to cope with the environment depend on the efficacy of the solutions that his culture provides, and the skills he develops are dependent on the adequacy of the preparatory institutions to which he has been exposed. To the extent that schools and informal types of preparation are inadequate to the tasks men face, social disruption and personal failure will be inevitable no matter how strong the individual's psychological capacities. Similarly, the kinds of motivation that people have and the directions in which such motivation will be channeled will depend on the incentive systems in a society—the patterns of behavior and performance that are valued and those that are condemned. Finally, the ability of persons to maintain psychological comfort will depend not only on their intrapsychic resources, but also—and perhaps more importantly—on the social supports available or absent in the environment. Men depend on others for justification and admiration, and few men can survive without support from some segment of their fellows (Mechanic 1970).

The foregoing is so obvious that I state these points with some embarrassment. As every introductory student of sociology learns in the first few weeks of his first course, solutions to life tasks become institutionalized and tend to be cumulative through the generations. Men learn through the experience of others, and solutions to environmental demands and challenges are taught from one generation to another. The ability of men and societies to adapt to the conditions of their lives depends in large part on the adequacy of such institutionalized solutions.

The influence of social structure is, of course, more complicated than this discussion suggests. The community not only defines solutions to environmental challenges, but also imposes new challenges through the social values it perpetuates. On the most primitive levels, the community defines territoriality, mobility, the pattern of fertility, food acquisition and use, mating, and social responsibility. But complex social structures also involve a large and varied set of demands that impinges on almost every aspect of life from survival to the most trivial of interrelationships.

Institutionalized solutions to environmental problems must change as the problems themselves change. To the extent that preparatory and evaluative institutions in a society are fitted to the types of problems people in the society must face, then most persons are likely to acquire the skills and capacities to meet life demands and challenges. But with rapid technological and social change, institutionalized solutions to new problems are likely to lag behind, and the probability increases that a larger proportion of the population will have difficulties in accommodating to life problems. In large part, the literature on stress and coping has aided the myth that adaptation is dependent on the ability of individuals to develop personal mastery over their environment. Indeed, most psychological studies of adaptation are studies of individuals and not of groups. But even a superficial thrust into the anthropological literature will make clear how interdependent men are even in the most simple of societies and how dependent they are on group solutions in dealing with environmental problems. Increasingly, it is clear that major stresses on modern man are not amenable to individual solutions, but depend on highly organized cooperative efforts that transcend those of any individual man no matter how well developed his personal resources.

The Influence of Social Networks on Adaptive Behavior

Although the stress literature often refers to group influences on adaptation to stress, such references are frequently diffuse and unenlightening.

Men relate to groups in a great variety of ways, and they may relate to the same group in different ways. Many groups define values and goals and serve as a reference point from which individuals may evaluate themselves. Or they may serve to encourage persons and help allay anxiety. But most important from the perspective of this paper is that group organization and cooperation allow for the development of mastery through specialization of function, pooling of resources and information, developing reciprocal help-giving relationships, and the like. It is a truism, but nevertheless important, that men are highly interdependent, and only through complex organization are the more complicated jobs of the community fulfilled. The effectiveness of individuals in many spheres of action is dependent almost exclusively on the maintenance of viable forms of organization and cooperation that allow important tasks to be mastered.

Much of the confusion in the stress literature results because stress is frequently seen as a short-term single stimulus rather than as a complex set of changing conditions that have a history and a future. Man must respond to these conditions through time and must adapt his behavior to the changing character of the stimuli. Thus mastery of stress is not a simple repertoire, but an active process over time in relationship to demands that are themselves changing, and that are often symbolically created by the groups within which man lives and new technologies which such groups develop. Adaptation itself creates new demands on man that require still further adaptations in a continuing spiral (Dubos 1965).

Moreover, many demands are ambiguous and intangible; they are created out of the social fabric and social climate that exist at any time. Challenges, therefore, are a product of the transaction between man and his environment, and many of the demands to which man must adapt are those that he has himself created. People to some extent can determine what demands they will be exposed to and at what pace. They can select from alternative environments and reference groups in testing themselves against their environments. They not only respond themselves, but require others to respond to them. This complex interplay between men involves adaptative techniques that are infrequently referred to in the study of short-term single stressors. Men pace themselves; they selectively seek information in relation to their needs for developing solutions on the one hand and for protecting their "selves" on the other; they anticipate future situations and plan solutions that they test; they frequently select the grounds on which their adaptive struggles will take place and carefully choose appropriate spheres of action. In short, they are more than seeds carried by the winds, or at least they can act as if they are.

One of the most impressive tests of the limits and potentialities of man's adaptive capacities occurs in those situations where men must live in controlled environments that are contrary to their values and goals, and where they are victims of arbitrary power, such as in concentration camps and prisons. We know from such situations that men often lose hope and become apathetic, accepting their fate without a fight. But we also know that even under the most desperate and unencouraging circumstances men succeed in developing competing forms of social organization that allow them to resist their oppressors and may allow survival under the most unpropitious of circumstances. Eugen Kogon (1958), a long-term resident of Buchenwald, describes the underground organization of inmates under the most hellish of conditions:

> There were a number of effective means by which the prisoners could assert their interests. They were all based on two essential prerequisites: power inside the camp, and a well-organized intelligence service. . . . Functional cohesion was insured by the prisoner intelligence service. Such a system was built up in every camp from the very outset. Reliable key members of the ruling group—or the group seeking power—were systematically wormed into all important posts, sometimes only after bitter and complex maneuvering. There they were able to observe everything that happened in the ranks of the SS and the prisoners, to obtain information on every personnel shift and policy trend, to overhear every conversation. . . . Every detail had its official "runners" ostensibly appointed in order to maintain liaison with the numerous scattered SS offices. Actually three-fourths of their time was taken up by work on behalf of the prisoners (pp. 254–255).

Kogon describes in detail how the underground organization was successful in controlling work assignments and reassignment of inmates to other camps and outside work details, and how they were successful in hiding and protecting valuable members of the underground from the SS. Kogon concedes that the prisoners were not strong enough to forestall general SS directives involving mass liquidations and similar actions, but they had vast influence on matters involving "the ordinary minutiae of camp life."

The type of organization which Kogon dramatically describes has been similarly observed in prisons (Sykes 1958; Sykes and Messinger 1960), mental hospitals (Goffman 1961, pp. 172–320), military organizations (Cohen 1966), and a great variety of other organizational contexts. To the extent that participants in organizations do not share the goals and values of its managers and authorities, an informal organization emerges that often impedes directives and programs that are seen as threatening to the welfare of organizational participants. I have described the principles underlying the power of such subordinate personnel elsewhere (Mechanic 1962a); let it suffice to note here that much of organizational power stems from small decisions made on daily tasks, or what Kogon refers to as "ordinary minutiae." Because higher-status organizational participants wish to be relieved of such burdensome "dirty work" or are dependent on others to perform it for other reasons, the dependency relationship and access to the performance of daily work give the subordinate considerable opportunity for effective vetoes on organizational policies.

As solutions to important problems become more complex, these problems are less likely to be resolved by individual initiative and action. In contrast, they are likely to depend on the ability of men to work out organized solutions involving group actions. It is within this context that it is necessary to note that individuals who may be adaptive and effective persons from a psychological perspective may be unfitted because of their values and individual orientations for the kinds of group cooperation that are necessary in developing solutions to particular kinds of community problems. Thus many effective copers may become impotent in influencing their environment because of their resistance or inability to submerge themselves into cooperative organized relationships with others.

It is not difficult to cite examples in modern life where men's disdain for organized participation interferes with effective performance. In the sphere of medicine, for example, the development of technology and associated growing costs of medical care require new forms of medical practice better fitted to the needs of the population than the highly individualized practice of medicine. Even in the absence of economic disincentives, doctors who are highly individualistic in their orientations tend to be reluctant to work within more organized practice settings (Mechanic 1968). Similarly in science, because of the costs and expansion of technology and specialized knowledge, team research is becoming more of a necessity. Yet, there are strong resistances to working cooperatively among many scientists who are highly individualistic and competitive in their orientations (Hagstrom 1965). Or to take another example, it is clear that organization of various aspects of the work force into groups that can bargain collectively is more effective than each man bargaining for himself. Although collective action is developing among a variety of professionals, in the higher professions there are very strong values that mitigate against collective action. To move more directly into the political realm, the futility of individual action in contesting such actions as the Vietnam war in contrast to collective opposition is evident. Group action is not necessarily effective, but it may provide at least a fighting chance.

In considering the conditions under which men will confront their environment, the symbolic aspects of threat and adaptation are extremely important. It is rarely the most oppressed who rise up to the challenges of their fate, but more usually those who have had a taste of the possibilities of improving their condition (Runciman 1966). Revolutions feed on faith and rarely occur when men see no way out. The unwillingness of many concentration camp victims to oppose their murderers may have, in part, resulted from the uncertainty of their individual fates, but more likely such efforts seemed futile and hopeless. In contrast, when men have hopes of success they are often willing to take on the most powerful of adversaries. This is, of course, all very speculative. Students of coping and adaptation would do well to invest greater attention to the question of how men see their environment and their own potency in meeting the challenges of that environment.

This brings me to consideration of a serious misconception that appears to run throughout the stress literature—the notion that successful adaptation requires an accurate perception of reality. There is perhaps no thought so stifling as to see ourselves in proper perspective. We all maintain our sense of self-respect and energy for action through perceptions that enhance our self-importance and self-esteem, and we maintain our sanity by suppressing the tremendous vulnerability we all experience in relation to the risks of the real world (Wolfenstein 1957). It is the beauty of symbolic environments that they allow men to enhance their sense of self-importance while permitting the community to persist at the same time. Most men tend to rate themselves and their qualities somewhat higher than their fellows would rate them, and the social contract among men allows each to control the definition of the situation to some extent on matters most close to his own self-interest. When the contract breaks down, one can usually locate groups that help sustain one's own self-definition, and social life is loosely enough organized so that most men can manage to sustain comforting self-perceptions.

The appropriate criterion for evaluating various defensive processes is the extent to which such defenses facilitate coping and mastery. Obviously, if defensive processes reach too far beyond what is acceptable to one's fellows, they create difficulty and interfere with successful adaptation. But many misperceptions of reality aid coping and mastery, energize involvement and participation in life endeavors, and alleviate pain and discomfort that would distract the person from successful efforts at mastery. Reality, of course, is a social construction, and to the extent that perspectives are shared and socially reinforced they may facilitate adaptation irrespective of their objective truth. It is well known that if men define situations as real, they are real in their consequences.

There are other concepts that have been taken up by psychologists who study stress that are probably more important to their own self-conceptions than they are for most people. A variable like "accessibility to self" may have some importance for introspective psychologists, but there is no good evidence that I know of that relates such variables to successful adaptation. In fact, there is some reason to believe that in many life endeavors too much self-awareness or introspection retards successful coping efforts. Many successful copers tend to be rather insensitive to their own intrapsychic experience and tend to orient themselves more to their outer environment than to their inner world (Korchin and Ruff 1964). Some very successful performers are truly public personalities in that they orient themselves outwardly and tend to have no very elaborate inner life. In contrast, there are persons who, by their abilities to see complexities in every issue, find it difficult to mobilize to attack any issue.

Some Problems in the Theory and Methodology of Stress Studies

If we take the position that adaptation is anticipatory as well as reactive and that men frequently approach their environment with plans, the study of such processes takes a somewhat different direction. Within such a view, man attempts to take on tasks he feels he can handle, he actively seeks information and feedback, he plans and anticipates problems, he insulates himself against defeat in a variety of ways, he keeps his options open, he distributes his commitments, he sets the stage for new efforts by practice and rehearsal, he tries various solutions, and so on. One cannot study such activities very effectively within an experimental mode that subjects man to specific stimuli and only measures limited reactions to these. But methodological models to successfully study such active processes of coping are very much undeveloped, and the lack of richness in the experimental stress literature reflects the lack of a successful experimental technology for studying adaptive attempts over time.

However much we may lament the fact, the development of fields of study follows the development of research technologies more than theoretical problems. In the stress field we have been the victim of many technologies that were useful and interesting in their own way, but that diverted researchers from basic issues. Perhaps most prominent have been the clinical interview and psychological assessment techniques popular among ego psychologists. The clinical interview depended too fully on retrospective reports, and the structure of such data in the absence of controls allowed each investigator to promote his favorite set of conceptions. Similarly, the use of personality assessment tools frequently allowed the investigator to explain, but not illuminate, performance differences. Thus we learned that men achieved because they had a need for achievement, that they were prejudiced because they were authoritarian, and that they did not participate in organizations because they were alienated. This form of absorption by naming took on the character of a popular sport, and although each of these conceptions involved an underlying theory of personality, the theory itself was either discredited or forgotten while the technologists continued to use the various measures that they could correlate with a host of other information. Because the study of stress has been to some extent limited by the fashionable methodologies of the past few decades, the picture of adaptation that emerges from the literature is one that depicts man as reactive and individualistic and his mode of coping as largely intrapsychic.

The major exception to this generalization has been the study of disasters and other real-life stresses under natural conditions. Approaches to natural stresses can follow a quasi-experimental design and, under some conditions, can utilize appropriate comparison groups. These studies for the most part present a much richer picture of the complexity of social adaptation and related factors. But given the complexity of such situations, it is often difficult to ferret out very precisely the variables most influential in modes of adaptation. The literature on social adaptation would benefit substantially from a richer interaction between field studies and more precise laboratory experiments, and more experimentation utilizing simulations of real situations. There are obvious ethical barriers in simulating stressful life circumstances, but there are many real circumstances that are amenable to study using experimental methodologies. Also, we have to develop more complex experimental models that do not restrict so closely the subject's opportunity to exercise his adaptive repertoire in dealing with laboratory situations. We must provide richer opportunities for subjects than the option of pushing one or another lever. Particularly impressive use of quasi-experimental models under natural circumstances are such investigations as the study by Epstein (1962) of paratrooper exercises and the Skipper and Leonard (1968) study of response to the stress of hospitalization and tonsillectomy.

It is likely that in the near future we have most to learn from field studies of adaptation to particular stress events over time. Such involvement requires greater emphasis on prospective and processual studies. Because this need has been expressed many times before, I will emphasize some more specific considerations rather than the more general points.

It is clear that we must go beyond people's subjective reports of how they feel and how they have responded to particular stressful circumstances. Such reports are particularly dubious when they describe events retrospectively, because we know that part of the process of adaptation involves the subtle restructuring of the individual's attitudinal set toward events that have taken place (Davis 1963; Robbins 1969). Successful adaptation requires changes in attitudes and perspectives that are sufficiently subtle so that the person hardly recognizes the changes himself. Large and sudden modifications of attitudes and perspectives are likely to produce new stresses, and, indeed, such large changes are themselves evidence of difficulties and disruptions in successful adaptation. We thus must be suspicious of reconstructions of the past as true representations of what really took place.

But even reports of events involving continuing activities and use of short recall periods may have dubious reliability. If we are not to throw the baby out with the bath water, we have to devote considerable effort to defining what kinds of reports are generally trustworthy and which ones are not. We can anticipate that persons will more reliably report their sex, age, family composition, and similar matters than they will their mental status, marital happiness, and like matters. Even when dealing with "harder" variables, persons frequently distort their responses, as women do, for example, in their tendency to underestimate their age, as very old people who tend to overestimate their age, and as many others who tend to report their age in round numbers. In contrast, reports on such variables as loneliness have very low test-retest reliability (Nefzger and Lilienfeld 1959). To some extent this is characteristic of all mood responses, which may widely vary from one day to another. Investigators, however, must be reasonably clear as to what degree of reliability of measures their studies require and the general range of reliability of varying measures they might utilize.

Take, for example, data dealing with people's reports of their use of medical services. Such data may or may not be worthy of collection, depending on the interests of the investigator and the research question he is asking. If the investigator wishes to know whether a person has been to a dentist, a doctor, or has been hospitalized during the preceding year, respondent reports will provide a reasonably reliable approximation. If, for some reason, small differences in utilization of medical services are important to the study, then it is reasonably clear that respondent reports will be too biased to be of any use (Mechanic and Newton 1965). Similarly, if an investigator wishes to note no more than crude differences between social categories on some measure of utilization, respondent reports will serve his purpose more than if he wishes to assign specific reliable scores to individual persons. Even in the case of more crude analyses of such data, respondent reports are likely to be unacceptable if there is reason to believe that there are systematic biases in reporting among different social groups.

Reports on such matters as having a heart condition, undergoing surgery, being hospitalized, and going to a doctor are reasonably "hard" in that these situations will have required specific actions on the part of the respondent that are not routine. But most studies of stress involve questions about very ordinary things that concern routine behavior and common attitudes, and such data are particularly suspect. For example, in family studies when identical questions are asked of husband and wife concerning routine activities in the family, husband-wife correlations are very small (Brown and Rutter 1966). Similarly, we know, for example, that what mothers tell you about themselves and what they tell you about the behavior of their children tend to be more highly correlated than data obtained independently from mother and child (Mechanic 1964). Too frequently investigators end up studying subjects' tendencies to respond and little else.

It is extraordinary that there are so few attempts to obtain independent data on behavior, because it is often accessible to research investigators willing to put in a little effort. It is possible, for example, to obtain medical and other records that allow some assessment of the value of what people tell you. These records, of course, have their own sources of unreliability, but investigators are on much firmer ground if they have both respondent and record data available to them. We need, in general, further development of behavior ratings that are likely to depict the variables we are really interested in more satisfactorily than do the measures more ordinarily used. This is no simple task, but it is one we will have to take on at some point. Those who deceive themselves that in the future we will develop some simple paper-and-pencil test to measure coping or adaptive potentialities are bound to be disillusioned; for the concern we face is so complex and multifaceted that it should be apparent that when we do develop some adequate measures, they are likely to be very complex ones. My own view is that such measures will have to be in the form of behavioral tests, and that the ordinary paper-and-pencil tests are incapable of the task.

At the theoretical level, one of the largest tasks that stress researchers face is the development of models that specify in a predictive sense under what conditions one set of adaptations will develop in contrast to some other set. If the study of adaptation is to develop as a theoretical area, then we must do more than describe the array of behaviors characteristic of persons' adaptive attempts; we must begin to specify the relative probabilities that, under given circumstances, one coping attempt will follow rather than another. This theoretical approach will depend on rich field studies that depict the scope of alternatives, followed by more controlled laboratory studies that attempt to determine the conditions under which one or another form of behavior follows. In short, theoretical needs require a range of methods, and if investigators do not choose to be eclectic themselves, at least some dialogue among approaches must be maintained.

One is beginning to see a more sophisticated theoretical approach emerging from this kind of interaction. It is promising, for example, that experimentalists who previously took the view that people avoided "discomforting information" are now more appreciative that sometimes they do and sometimes they do not and that the entire matter is more complicated than earlier views suggested (Freedman and Sears 1965). It may be too early to suggest convergences, but it may be that persons seek out information contrary to their views and perspectives when such information is important to their future coping efforts; discomforting information may primarily be avoided when it is believed to be of little utility. Or to take another example, early studies were concerned with the simplistic question as to whether or not high interactors were more or less successful at various tasks. There is a growing appreciation of not only the fact that there are different kinds of interaction (which I previously referred to as interaction for instrumental purposes and interaction for the purposes of support), but also that interaction may not only facilitate activity and support people, but also arouse competition and anxiety and lead to interference with effective performance (Hall 1969; Mechanic 1962b). Such variables as rate of interaction are too crude to be informative theoretically in understanding adaptation.

It is encouraging that social psychologists in general are moving away from using their concepts to absorb existing data and are giving increasing efforts to developing an understanding of the contingencies affecting behavior. For example, when dissonance theory (Festinger 1957) first became fashionable it was frequently used to explain the results of a variety of studies by citing a dissonance explanation. Recently, however, there have been more serious attempts to specify on the basis of various contingencies the likely route of dissonance reduction. Similar efforts are taking place in the study of social comparison processes. It has been very common for social scientists to explain data after the fact by arguing that a person's behavior was a result of choosing particular reference groups. The more interesting issue—and one now receiving more attention—concerns the conditions under which identification with various possible reference groups occurs. Ego psychology has similarly been handicapped by the failure to specify in any rigorous way the conditions under which one set of defenses will occur in opposition to another mode of adaptation, and under what conditions particular defenses will be selected. The literature abounds with discussions of particular defenses in isolation from others. Thus we find discussions dealing with compensation (that is, the tendency to do particularly well in some areas to overcome inadequacies in others) without awareness of a literature on status congruency (the psychological tendency to maintain one's various statuses at approximately the same level), which appears in opposition to it. The theory of compensation argues that people strive toward maintaining unequal levels of performance, while the theory of status congruency maintains that people strive toward maintaining equal levels of performance. Such contradictions lead to theoretical contributions in that they suggest that important intervening variables have been neglected. In the example cited it is likely that people tend to compensate when a particular dimension of their status or performance is blocked or unalterable. However, when there is opportunity to perform in any of several spheres, it may be that the need for congruency is dominant. I know of no specific data that clearly resolve the contradiction, but the recognition of a contradiction raises new issues.

In conclusion, I think that it would be advisable to pursue studies of adaptation with two particular models in mind. (1) On the one hand, we need more emphasis on field studies of adaptive struggles over time. Further attention must be given to collecting data at various points in time in contrast to using retrospective reports. Moreover, such studies should give greater emphasis to the development of behavioral measures. (2) At the same time, we should be pursuing a variety of cross-sectional studies that link particular adaptive strategies and coping devices to effective behavior on a variety of life tasks. Although there are many studies of a cross-sectional nature in the stress area, few are concerned with the relationship between what people do and how effective they are. In the past, more than a reasonable proportion of the total research effort has gone into attempts to link personality traits with effectiveness, and in many ways this has been a disappointing effort. My guess is that greater emphasis on coping strategies themselves will provide a greater payoff. Finally, I believe that a field has the greatest payoff when there is constant interplay between studies in natural settings and more precise experimental investigation. We should do all we can to nurture those bridges that make such collaboration possible and fruitful.

References

Brown, G., and Rutter, M. The measurement of family activities and relationships. *Human relations,* 1966, 19, 241–263.

Cohen, A. *Deviance and control.* Englewood Cliffs, N.J.: Prentice-Hall, 1966.

Davis, F. *Passage through crisis: Polio victims and their families.* Indianapolis: Bobbs-Merrill, 1963.

Dubos, R. *Man adapting.* New Haven, Conn.: Yale University Press, 1965.

Epstein, S. The measurement of drive and conflict in humans. In M. R. Jones, ed., *Nebraska symposium on motivation.* Lincoln, Neb.: University of Nebraska Press, 1962.

Festinger, L. *A theory of cognitive dissonance.* Evanston, Ill.: Row Peterson, 1957.

Freedman, J., and Sears, D. Selective exposure. In L. Berkowitz, ed., *Advances in experimental social psychology,* vol. 2. New York: Academic Press, 1965.

Goffman, E. *Asylums* New York: Doubleday, 1961.

Hagstrom, W. *The scientific community.* New York: Basic Books, 1965.

Hall, D. The impact of peer interaction during an academic role transition. *Sociology of Education*, 1969, 42(2), 118–140.

Kogon, E. *The theory and practice of bell.* New York: Berkeley Medallion Books, 1958.

Korchin, S., and Ruff, G. Personality characteristics of the Mercury astronauts. In G. H. Grosser, H. Wechsler, and M. Greenblatt, eds., *The threat of impending disaster: Contributions to the psychology of stress.* Cambridge, Mass.: M.I.T. Press, 1964.

McGrath, J., ed. *Social and psychological factors in stress.* New York: Holt, Rinehart & Winston, 1970.

Mechanic, D. Sources of power of lower participants in complex organizations. *Administrative Science Quarterly*, 1962a, 7, 349–364.

———. *Students under stress.* New York: Free Press, 1962b.

———. The influence of mothers on their children's health attitudes and behavior. *Pediatrics*, 1964, 33, 444–453.

———. General medical practice in England and Wales. *New England Journal of Medicine*, 1968, 279, 680–689.

———. Some problems in developing a social psychology of adaptation to stress. In J. McGrath, ed., *Social and psychological factors in stress.* New York: Holt, Rinehart & Winston, 1970.

Mechanic, D., and Newton, M. Some problems in the analysis of morbidity data. *Journal of Chronic Disease*, 1965, 18, 569–580.

Nefzger, N., and Lilienfeld, A. Item reliability and related factors in a community survey of emotionality. *Sociometry*, 1959, 22, 236–246.

Robbins, L. Follow-up studies of behavior disorders in children. Paper presented to the W.P.A.-R.M.P.A. Symposium on Psychiatric Epidemiology, University of Aberdeen, July 1969.

Runciman, W. G. *Relative deprivation and social justice.* Berkeley and Los Angeles: University of California Press, 1966.

Skipper, J. K., Jr., and Leonard R. C. Children, stress and hospitalization: A field experiment. *Journal of Health and Social Behavior*, 1968, 9, 275–287.

Sykes, G. *The society of captives.* Princeton, N.J.: Princeton University Press, 1958.

Sykes, G., and Messinger, S. The inmate social system. In R. Cloward et al., eds., *Theoretical studies in social organization of the prison.* New York: Social Science Research Council, 1960.

Wolfstein, M. *Disaster: A psychological essay.* New York: Free Press, 1957.

7

Social Psychologic Factors Affecting the
Presentation of Bodily Complaints

Patients often recognize symptoms for which they seek medical assistance, but, on the basis of a history and physical and laboratory examination, the physician cannot obtain evidence to account for or justify the patients' complaints.[1] Such patients conform in part to Gillespie's concept of hypochondria, which he viewed as "a persistent preoccupation with the bodily health, out of proportion to any existing justification and with a conviction of disease."[2] There is considerable disagreement, however, on the appropriate formal definition of hypochondria,[3] and it may be incorrect to apply the same designation to profound and persistent hypochondrical syndromes associated with psychiatric illness and the type of hypochondriasis commonly seen in general practice.

Perceptions of Symptoms

Estimates derived from British and American morbidity surveys indicate that three of four persons have symptoms in any given month for which they take some definable action such as use of medication, bed rest, consulting a physician and limiting activity.[4] In addition, persons experience many other symptoms, which they regard as trivial and which they ignore. Investigators believe that it is pointless to attempt to measure symptoms that do not receive some type of treatment or special attention since they occur commonly and have too little impact to be reported accurately in household surveys.[5,6] Yet such symptoms overlap appreciably with typical presenting complaints among patients seeking medical care.[7]

The major task of this paper is to suggest how normal attribution processes develop in the definition of symptoms. As an initial formulation, it appears that persons tend to notice bodily sensations when they depart from more ordinary feelings. Each person tends to appraise new bodily perceptions against prior experience and his anticipations based on the experiences of others and on general knowledge. Many symptoms occur so commonly throughout life that they become part of ordinary expectations and are experienced as normal variations. Other experiences, such as a young girl's first menstruation, might be extremely frightening if prior social learning has not occurred, but would ordinarily be accepted as normal if it had. In analyzing responses to more unusual symptoms it is instructive to examine situations in which normal attribution processes become disrupted as a consequence of special kinds of learning, and in this regard hypochondriasis among medical students is an interesting example.

The Case of the Medical Student

It has frequently been observed that medical students experience symptom complexes that they ascribe to some pathologic process. This syndrome appears to have high prevalence—approximately 70 per cent.[8,9] Factors contributing to the development of this syndrome usually include social stress and anxiety, bodily symptoms and detailed but incomplete information on a disease involving symptoms similar to the bodily indications perceived by the student. Hunter, Lohrenz and Schwartzman describe the process as follows:

> The following constellation of factors occur regularly. The student is under internal or external stress, such as guilt, fear of examinations and the like. He notices in himself some innocuous physiological or psychological dysfunction, e.g., extrasystoles, forgetfulness. He attaches to this an undeserved importance of a fearful kind usually modeled after some patient he has seen, clinical anecdote he has heard, or a member of his family who has been ill.[9]

It is not clear from such descriptions to what extent each of the components—stress, bodily symptoms and external cues—is necessary to the process and what specific role each plays. Since both stress and bodily symptoms are extremely common among students in general—and the phenomenon in question does not appear to occur so dramatically or with equal prevalence among them—it seems reasonable to suspect that the medical student's access to more detailed medical information contributes greatly to the attribution process.

An experiment by Schachter and Singer[10] helps explain how information affects emotional response. Subjects were told that the experimenters were interested in the effects of a vitamin compound called Suproxin (a nonexistent substance) on their vision, and these subjects were given an injection. Each subject was then asked to wait, while the drug took effect, in a room with another student who appeared to be a subject who had received the same injection, but who was really a confederate of the experimenter.

The injection received was epinephrine bitartrate (adrenaline), whereas subjects in control groups received a saline solution (the placebo). Some of the subjects who received epinephrine were told to anticipate heart pounding, hand tremor and a warm and flushed face; this group was correctly informed. A second group receiving epinephrine was given no information about what to expect; this group was called the ignorant group. A third group receiving epinephrine was incorrectly informed that their feet would feel numb, that they would have itching sensations, and that they would get a slight headache; this group was called the misinformed group. While the subject was waiting for the "experiment" to begin, the confederate of the experimenter went into a scheduled act in which he slowly worked himself into a "euphoric" state playing imaginary basketball, flying paper airplanes, hula-hooping, and so on. During this period the subject was observed behind a one-way window, and his behavior was rated in terms of relevant categories. Later, he was asked to report as well his subjective feelings. Three additional groups were studied in a variation of the same situation: another epinephrine informed group; an epinephrine ignorant group; and a placebo group. In this second situation the confederate simulated anger instead of euphoria. Thus, it is possible to assess the influences of epinephrine, the various expectations subjects are given for their bodily experiences, and the different environmental cues (i.e., an angry or euphoric confederate).

Subjects who received an injection of epinephrine and who had no correct or appropriate explanation of the side effects that they experienced (particularly the epinephrine misinformed group) were most affected in their behavior and feeling states by the cues provided by the student confederate. The nature of the emotion—whether anger or euphoria—was influenced by the behavior of the confederate. Schachter and Singer believe that emotion involves a two-stage process requiring physiologic arousal and a definition of it. They maintain that the same internal state can be labeled in a variety of ways, resulting in diferent emotional reactions. External influences on definitions of internal states are particularly important when persons lack an appropriate explanation of what they are experiencing.

With the use of the Schachter-Singer formulation, "medical students' disease" can be characterized as follows: Medical school exposes students to continuing stress resulting from the rapid pace, examinations, anxieties in dealing with new clinical experiences and the like. Students, thus, are emotionally aroused with some frequency, and like others in the population, they experience a high prevalence of transient symptoms. The exposure to specific knowledge about disease provides the student with a new framework for identifying and giving meaning to previously neglected bodily feelings. Diffuse and ambiguous symptoms regarded as normal in the past may be reconceptualized within the context of newly acquired knowledge of disease. Existing social stress may heighten bodily sensations through autonomic activation, making the student more aware of his bodily state, and motivating him to account for what he is experiencing. The new information that the student may have about possible disease and the similarity between the symptoms of a particular condition and his own symptoms establishes a link that he would have more difficulty making if he were less informed. Moreover, the student—in the process of acquiring new medical information—may begin to pay greater attention to his own bodily experiences and may also attempt to imagine how certain symptoms feel. This tendency to give attention to bodily feelings may assist the development of the syndrome.

Woods, Natterson and Silverman[8] found that, contrary to usual belief, "medical students' disease" was not an isolated experience linked to a particular aspect of medical training, but occurred with relatively equal frequency throughout the four years of medical school. Thus, the syndrome's occurrence may depend on the coincidental existence of student arousal, the presence of particular bodily feelings, and cues acquired from new information about disease that seems relevant to existing symptoms.

Hunter, Lohrenz and Schwartzman,[9] on the basis of their study, conclude that symptom choice is influenced by "a variety of accidental, historical and learning factors, in which the mechanism of identification plays a major role." Yet there appears to be a variety of factors that may increase the probability of the occurrence of the syndrome, and it is important to inquire under what conditions concern about illness in contrast to alternative definitions will become manifest. The normal person may have a variety of symptoms without experiencing a fear of illness. Many investigators of hypochondriacal patients note that reported symptoms tend to be diffuse and may change from one occasion to another. Such patients often report numerous complaints referring to a variety of organ systems, or they report nonlocalized symptoms: insomnia, itching, dizziness, weakness, lack of energy, pain all over, nausea, and the like.[11-13] Kenyon,[14] in reviewing 512 patient case records at the Bethlem Royal and Maudsley hospitals, found that the head and neck, abdomen and chest were the regions of the body most frequently affected, and that the most typical complaints were headache and gastrointestinal and musculoskeletal symptoms. Striking features of almost all descriptions of hypochondriacal patients, particularly in early stages, are the lack of specificity of complaint and similarity to frequently occurring symptoms in normal populations. Moreover, many of the complaints tend to be of symptoms that commonly occur under stress and that epidemiologic studies show to have very high prevalence in ordinary community populations.[15,16] The common occurrence of such symptoms and their diffuseness establish conditions under which widely varying attributions may reasonably occur. Incorrect attributions may occur as well in existing organic disease because of the diffuseness of symptoms, referred pain, particular characteristics of the patient or some combination of these factors.

It is noteworthy that "medical students' disease" terminates readily and within a relatively short time. Woods and his colleagues report that the syndrome sometimes disappears spontaneously, but more often through further study of the illness or by direct or covert consultation with an instructor or physician. They suggest that it is "reassurance" that limits the condition, but the term is exceedingly vague and has a variety of meanings. Most reports in the literature concerning more persistent hypochondria suggest that such patients are not easily reassured, and thus it would be useful to have more specific understanding of the mechanism by which "medical students' disease" is short-circuited.

One way in which the medical student discovers errors in attribution is through further understanding of diagnostics. As he learns more about the disease, he may discover that the attribution he made does not really fit or that a great variety of symptoms that commonly occur may be characteristic of the clinical picture. Another possibility is that the stress in the student's life that is fluctuating subsides with some relief in his anxiety, and his awareness of his symptoms may decline. How the incorrect attribution comes to be corrected has never been studied, but possibly the student's growing knowledge of symptomatology sharpens his judgment about his own complaints. If clear knowledge is indeed necessary to disconfirm the attribution adequately, the syndrome should be more persistent when knowledge is disputed and uncertain. In this light it is of interest that "medical students' disease" of a psychiatric character appears to be less transient and more chronic than such syndromes that develop around fears of physical illness.[8] In the psychiatric area it is more difficult to separate the attribution from the entity to which the attribution is made.

Another issue concerns the origins of the initial attribution of illness. The conclusion reached by Hunter, Lohrenz and Schwartzman[9] that identification plays a major part has already been noted, and this appears to be the most generally accepted psychiatric point of view. The concept of identification as used by the authors in this respect is more descriptive than explanatory, and it encompasses the observation often made that the patient will frequently focus on a disease that affected a loved one. An examination of cases described in the literature suggests that the localization and definition of the complaint may depend on idiosyncrasies or may be fortuitous. Ladee[3] reports the observation of Orbán concerning a veterinary surgeon who felt a pain in the right lower part of his abdomen. Apparently, he feared an incipient bowel obstruction rather than appendicitis, and Ladee explains that appendicitis is rare among cattle whereas ileus is frequent. Felix Brown,[17] in a thoughtful review of 41 cases of hypochondria, notes the important influence of topical suggestions. Many commentators have also observed how frequently symptoms of a particular kind follow publicity given to the illness or death of a well known personality or a dramatic mass-media demonstration concerning some disease.

It appears that the concept of identification may be too diffuse and imprecise in encompassing such varied phenomena as the association between mother and child, audience and public figure, and the occurrence of a stomach pain and seeing a movie concerning a person with stomach cancer. An alternative perspective from which to analyze such influences would involve consideration of factors affecting the perception of personal vulnerability.

Perceptions of Personal Vulnerability

Although persons may vary widely in their sense of invulnerability—which appears to be linked with their levels of self-esteem—psychologic survival generally depends on the ability of people to protect themselves from anxieties and fears involving low-risk occurrences to which all persons are exposed or dangers that they are powerless to prevent.[18,19] Feelings of invulnerability are threatened under circumstances of greatly increased risk such as combat and new and difficult experiences, but even under these conditions, persons generally manage to maintain a relatively strong sense of invulnerability through various psychologic defense processes and coping actions. However, a "near-miss" can dramatically undermine one's sense of invulnerability and may lead to extreme anxiety and fear reactions. The death of a close friend or co-worker in combat,[20] being involved in an automobile accident in which others are killed or suffer bodily injury, and learning that someone who is defined as having comparable ability to oneself has failed an important examination that one is intending to take[21] serve to threaten the sense of security.

Basic to the undermining of a sense of invulnerability are social comparison processes. It is much less difficult to explain injury to people of unlike characteristics without threat to oneself in that one can attribute the injury to aspects of the person that are different from one's own. When such persons are more like oneself—in terms of age, sex, life style or routine—it is much more difficult not to perceive oneself at risk, and personal intimacy or physical proximity similarly increases feelings of vulnerability.

Various studies suggest that self-esteem is an intervening variable between situation and response. Although the role of self-esteem is not fully clear, one possibility is that persons with high self-esteem see themselves as more capable of dealing with threatening situations and, thus, are less vulnerable.[22] The awareness that one is able to cope and that one has had success in the past in dealing with adversity insulates the person from anxiety.[23] This concept of the self-esteem effect appears most reasonable in cases in which coping ability can affect the situation and realistically reduce threat; it is not so obvious that self-esteem reduces a sense of threat of impending illness, although many writers on hypochondria note specifically that low self-esteem is associated with this syndrome. A sense of confidence may generalize to situations even when it is not particularly realistic, or may lead persons to focus less on bodily indications. This is clearly an area for more focused inquiry.

Some symptoms present in a fashion that makes them difficult to ignore, and many symptoms are sufficiently impressive in their occurrence or sufficiently disruptive of normal functioning so that variation in response is relatively limited. Moreover, many symptoms occur so as not to allow alternative attributions readily. Hypochondria developing around a fear that one has a fractured leg or an extremely high fever is not found ordinarily; indeed, the response to such symptoms is not mediated in any influential way by social and cultural variables. But when symptoms are more diffuse, variation in response is more likely to occur.

In sum, it has been maintained that most ordinarily occurring symptoms are considered normal or explained in conventional frameworks, as when muscle aches are attributed to unaccustomed physical activity or indigestion to overeating. When such ordinary symptoms occur concomitantly with emotional arousal, and when they are not easily explained within conventional and commonly available understandings, external cues become important in defining the character and importance of such bodily feelings. Such cues may be fortuitous, or they may be the consequence of prior experience, cultural learning or personal need for secondary gain. The manner in which sociocultural and psychologic contexts condition attributional responses requires further examination.

Social and Cultural Influences on Response to Symptoms

From very young ages children more or less learn to respond to various symptoms and feelings in terms of reactions of others to their behavior and social expectations in general. As children begin to mature, clear age and sex patterns become apparent, and the children become clearly differentiated in the manner in which they respond to pain, their risk-taking activities, and their readiness to express their apprehensions and hurts.[24] Learning influences the tendency of males as compared with females to take more risks, to seek medical care less readily, and to be less expressive about illness and appear more stoical.

The role of cultural differences in identification and response to illness has been described nicely by Zborowski[25] and has been amplified in a variety of other studies.[26] Zborowski, in studying reactions to pain in a New York City hospital among various ethnic groups, noted that whereas Jewish and Italian patients responded to pain in an emotional fashion, "Old Americans" were more stoical and "objective," and Irish more frequently denied pain. He also noted a difference in the attitude underlying Italian and Jewish concern about pain; although the Italian patients primarily sought relief from pain and were relatively satisfied when such relief was obtained, the Jewish patients appeared to be concerned mainly with the meaning of their pain and the consequences of pain for their future health and welfare. Thus, different attributional processes appeared to form the basis of these manifest similarities. Zborowski reported that Italian patients seemed relieved when they were given medication for pain, and their complaining ceased. In contrast, Jewish patients were reluctant to accept medication and appeared to have greater concern with the implications of their pain experience for their future health.

Other studies have similarly found that ethnic groups differentially report symptoms and seek medical assistance for them, and vary in the extent to which they are willing to accept psychologic interpretations of their complaints.[27,28] It is unclear whether the ethnic differences, noted in the literature, are a result of the fact that children with particular prior experiences and upbringing come to have more objective symptoms, interpret the same symptoms differently, express their concerns and seek help with greater willingness, or use a different vocabulary for expressing distress. Such distinctions are important.

Responses to Perceived Illness and Vocabularies of Distress

It is apparent that social learning will affect the vocabularies persons use to define their complaints and their orientations to seeking various kinds of care. It is reasonable to expect that persons from origins where the expression of symptoms and seeking help is permissible and encouraged will be more likely to do so, particularly under stressful circumstances. In contrast, in cultural contexts where complaining is discouraged, persons experiencing distress may seek a variety of alternative means for dealing with their difficulties. Zborowski, in describing the "Old American" family, stressed the tendency of the mother to teach the child to take pain "like a man," not to be a sissy and not to cry. Such training, according to Zborowski, does not discourage use of the doctor, but it implies that such use will be based on physical needs rather than on emotional concerns. One might, therefore, anticipate that persons with such backgrounds might be reluctant to express psychologic distress directly, but might express such distress through the presentation of physical complaints. Kerckhoff and Back,[29] in a study of the diffusion of a hysterical illness among female employees of a Southern mill alleged to be caused by an unknown insect, found that the prevalence of the condition was high among women under strain who could not admit they had a problem and who did not know how to cope with it.

Pauline Bart,[30] in comparing women who entered a neurology service, but who were discharged with psychiatric diagnoses, with women entering a psychiatric service of the same hospital, found them to be less educated, more rural, of lower socioeconomic status, and less likely to be Jewish than those who came directly to a psychiatric service. Bart suggests that these two groups of women were differentiated by their vocabularies of discomfort, which affected the manner in which they presented themselves. She also observed that 52 per cent on the psychiatric patients on the neurology service had had a hysterectomy as compared with only 21 per cent on the psychiatric service. The findings suggest that such patients may be expressing psychologic distress through physical attributions and, thus, expose themselves to a variety of unnecessary medical procedures.

Most of the understanding of the patient's complaint comes from observation of that part of the process that brings the patient into contact with the physician. It should be clear that this tends to focus on only a segment of the entire sample and excludes patients with comparable problems who do not seek assistance. Various analysts of the medical consultation, such as Balint,[31] note that the symptoms that the patient presents are frequently of no special consequence, but serve to establish a legitimate relation between patient and doctor. He maintains that the presentation of somatic complaints often masks an underlying emotional problem that is frequently the major reason the patient has sought help. Certainly, a complaint of illness may be one way of seeking reassurance and support through a recognized and socially acceptable relation when it is difficult for the patient to present the underlying problem in an undisguised form without displaying weaknesses and vulnerabilities contrary to expected and learned behavior patterns. The emphasis that Balint places on the symptom as a front for underlying emotional distress, although characteristic of some patients, neglects the fact that many patients who are more receptive to psychologic vocabularies may also be viewed as hypochondriacal.

The response to bodily indications may also depend on the social acceptability of certain types of complaints, and even the nature and site of the complaint, according to Balint, is a matter frequently negotiated between patient and physician. Harold Wolff[32] has also noted that minor pains from certain parts of the body may be more frequent because they are culturally more acceptable and because they bring greater sympathetic response. Hes,[33] in a study of hypochrondriac patients, referred to a psychiatric outpatient clinic, noted the inhibition of emotional expression as a result of culturally determined taboos on complaining about one's fate and a culturally determined excessive use of bodily language. He found these conditions particularly characteristic of Oriental Jewish women, who made up a major proportion of his patients with hypochondria.

Mechanic and Volkart[34] examined the influence of stress and inclination to use medical facilities among 600 male students at a major university. Stress (as measured by indexes of loneliness and nervousness) and inclination to use medical facilities (as measured by anticipated behavior given hypothetical illness situations) were clearly related to the use of a college health service during a one-year period. Among students with high stress and a high inclination to use medical facilities 73 per cent were frequent users of medical facilities (three or more times during the year), but among the low-inclination-low-stress group, only 30 per cent were frequent users of such services. Among those of high inclination, "stress" was an important influence in bringing people to the physician. Seventy-three per cent of persons experiencing high stress used facilities frequently, although only 46 per cent did so among those with low stress.[35] A similar trend was observed among those who were less inclined to seek advice from a doctor, but the relation between stress and actually seeking advice was substantially smaller and not statistically significant. These data support the interpretation that stress leads to an attempt to cope; those who are receptive to the patient role tend to adopt this particular mode of coping more frequently than those who are not so receptive. The previous discussion also suggests that when stress helps initiate a medical contact, the contact may be presented through a vocabulary of physical symptoms that frequently impress the physician as trivial or unimportant. A very similar study was carried out with comparable results among British women using two general-practice panels within the English National Health Service.[36]

The impression emerging from these studies is that there are at least two major patterns of behavior that physicians tend to regard as hypochondriacal. The first consists of patients who have a high inclination to use medical facilities and a willingness to use a vocabulary of psychologic distress, openly complaining of unhappiness, frustration and dissatisfaction.[37] The more common and difficult patient to deal with is one who has a high receptivity to medical care but who lacks a vocabulary of psychologic distress. Such patients tend to present the doctor with a variety of diffuse physical complaints for which he can find no clear-cut explanation, but he cannot be sure that they do not indeed suffer from some physical disorder that he has failed to diagnose.

Patients who express psychologic distress through a physical language tend to be uneducated or to come from cultural groups where the expression of emotional distress is inhibited. Such patients frequently face serious life difficulties and social stress, but the subculture within which they function does not allow legitimate expression of their suffering nor are others attentive to their pleas for support when they are made. Because of their experiences these patients frequently feel, sometimes consciously but more frequently on a level of less than full awareness, that expression of their difficulties is a sign of weakness and will be deprecated. They thus dwell on bodily complaints, some that are ever present, and others that are concomitant with their experience of emotional distress. These patients are often elderly, lonely and insecure, and they may be inactive enough to have time to dwell on their difficulties. When such patients seek out physicians they may use their physical symptoms and complaints as a plea for help.

Effects of Emotional Distress on Symptoms

It has been suggested at various points that emotional arousal appears to heighten the experience of symptoms, and in this regard the literature on reactions to pain is noteworthy. Beecher[38] has reported the failure of 15 different research groups to establish any dependable effects of even large doses of morphine on pain of experimental origin in man. He has found it necessary to distinguish between pain as an original sensation and pain as a psychic reaction. As Beecher notes, one of the difficulties with most forms of laboratory pain is that they minimize the psychic reaction, which has an essential role in pain associated with illness. For example, in a comparative study he found that civilian patients undergoing surgery reported strikingly more frequent and severe pain than wounded soldiers with greater tissue trauma. He observed that such variations resulted from varying subjective definitions, and concluded that there is no simple, direct relation between the wound per se and the pain experienced.

A variety of reports both of an anthropologic nature and in the experimental literature indicate how a person's definition of a painful experience conditions how much pain he is willing to tolerate and what he will endure without protest. In experimental situations persons can be given instructions and incentives to endure severe pain stimulation.[39,40,41] Here it is difficult to separate what people may feel from their willingness to control expression patterns, but many such reports suggest that when there is strong positive motivation, people will undergo extraordinary pain without complaint. Also, if intensely involved in some patterns of behavior, they may not become immediately aware of severe body trauma.[42]

The reactive component in illness has long been recognized as an important aspect not only in defining the condition but also in the patient's response to treatment and in the course of the illness. Imboden and his colleagues have studied prolonged convalescence in chronic brucellosis and influenza, in which they argue that emotional stress concomitant with the course of the illness may become intermingled with symptoms of the illness in such a way that the end point of the illness becomes confused with continuing emotional distress.[43,44] They note that symptoms of emotional distress may be attributed to the physical illness well beyond the normal course of the infection, which may serve to maintain the patient's self-concept.

The studies on prolonged convalescence suggest some of the conditions under which misattribution may occur. For example, the course of influenza and brucellosis is likely to leave the patient fatigued, with a lack of energy and interest, weakness and a variety of other somatic symptoms. These symptoms may also accompany depression and other emotional distress. The similarity in the symptoms makes it reasonable for the patient to attribute these symptoms after the illness to the persistence of the illness. The similarity that makes the errors of attribution more likely also makes it difficult for the physician to determine when the symptoms are a product of an emotional problem and when they are complications of the physical illness. Thus, the physician may unwittingly reinforce the patient's confusion.

The manner in which physicians may come to reinforce particular patient tendencies is suggested by a variety of reports.[45,46] Zola,[45] for example, on the basis of a study of patients for whom no medical disease was found, suggests that the patient's cultural background influenced how he presented his symptoms and, thus, how the doctor evaluated them. Although the ethnic groups studied did not differ in the extent of their life difficulties, Italians, who are more emotional in the presentation of symp-toms and give more attention and expression to pain and distress, were more likely to be evaluated as suffering from a psychogenic condition.

Treating the Chronic Complainer—Correcting Errors in Attribution

In a classic paper, Felix Brown[17] defined bodily complaints in five ways: partly on a physiologic or somatic level, associated with anxiety; symbolic of something else; consistent with mood disturbance, usually depression; by substitution or conversion of an affect, usually anxiety, with more or less elimination of the affect; and with more or less conscious purpose for the patient—purposive hypochondriasis.

The first three groups are most typical of the chronic complainer seen in ordinary medical practice. Ordinarily, it is believed that doctors must provide general reassurance, which relieves the patient's level of distress, but if the implications of some of the theoretical statements made earlier are followed, it should become clear why reassurance alone may not be the most effective approach. Frequently, the interpretation that the patient has made of his symptoms is a provisional and vague definition, and, as Balint indicates, this attribution is readily changed by the physician's suggestions. The physician may be able to alleviate the patient's distress to the extent that he can provide the patient with benign interpretations of his distress that are credible and to the extent to which he can reassure him and bolster his esteem and sense of mastery. To provide general reassurance alone may have no effect on the patient's perspective relevant to the meaning of his symptoms, although it may contribute to the alleviation of anxiety. Providing alternative attributions is difficult because they not only must relieve anxiety but also must be culturally and psycho-logically acceptable to the patient as well. For example, if the patient has learned that a psychologic expression of distress is unacceptable, such an interpretation by the physician may be of little use to the patient, may exacerbate his anxiety, and may disrupt the relation between doctor and patient.

The suggestion that the attribution the doctor provides must be credible means that it must be consistent with what the patient is experiencing and likely to experience in the future. If not, it may serve to arouse the patient's anxiety further and will not be taken seriously. Some evidence on this matter comes from a study of Rickels and his colleagues[47,48] on the effects of placebos. Suggestibility is an important factor in the medical situation, and placebos have been found to alleviate distress in a wide range of medical disorders.[26] Rickels and his colleagues, however, found that patients with prolonged experience with anxiety and the use of tranquilizing drugs do poorly when treated by placebos, and many suffer a worsening of their anxiety state. Patients who are attuned to their inner feelings and have had experiences with psychoactive drugs do not experience placebos as credible. The impact of the suggestion effect is hardly equal to the patients' past experiences of true relief of their symptoms with tranquilizers, and the failure of the placebo to reduce their anxieties to the level they expect may alarm them and make them think that they are more upset than usual.

Such an interpretation is offered by Storms and Nisbett[49] in a study of insomniac subjects. These subjects were given placebos to take before going to bed; some were told that the pill would increase their arousal, and others that it would decrease it. The former reported that they got to sleep more quickly than previously, whereas the latter reported that they took longer to get to sleep than before. Storms and Nisbett believe that the subjects who thought that their arousal was due to the pill felt less upset and could fall asleep more easily, but those who continued to feel arousal despite the fact that the pill was to reduce their arousal defined themselves as particularly upset. Although caution is required in generalizing to clinical situations, such studies illustrate how the efficacy of the doctor's interpretations of his patient's problems will depend on the extent to which they are credible in terms of the patient's experiences and the extent to which he anticipates the patient's reactions to symptoms and treatment.

The adequacy of the doctor's management of the patient is also likely to depend on the kinds of expectations and instructions he provides the patient in preparation for what lies ahead. Whether doctors say anything or not, patients will anticipate and acquire expectations of the course of their condition, how they expect to feel, what is likely to happen and the like. To the extent that the patient is not instructed, his expectations may be highly contrary to what is likely to occur, and this discrepancy may alarm the patient and disrupt his management. Various experimental studies suggest that very modest instruction and information have an important effect on patient outcomes,[50,51] and on facilitating preventive health actions.[22]

Egbert and his colleagues,[50] for example, selected a random group of patients undergoing surgery and gave them simple information, encouragement and instruction concerning the impending operation and means of alleviating postoperative pain. The researchers, however, were not involved in the medical care of the patients studied, and they did not participate in decisions concerning them. An independent evaluation of the postoperative period and the length of stay of patients in the experimental and control groups showed that communication and instruction had an important beneficial effect.

In a similar experimental study by Skipper and Leonard,[51] children admitted to a hospital for tonsillectomy were randomized into experimental and control groups. In the experimental group patients and their mothers were admitted to the hospital by a specially trained nurse, who attempted to create an atmosphere that would facilitate the communication of information to the mother and increase her freedom to verbalize her anxieties. Mothers were told what routine events to expect and when they were likely to occur, including the actual time schedule for the operation. The investigators found that the emotional support reduced the mothers' stress and changed their definition of the hospital situation, which in turn had a beneficial effect on their children. Children in the experimental group experienced smaller changes in blood pressure, temperature and other physiologic measures; they were less likely to suffer from postoperative emesis and made a better adaptation to the hospital, and they made a more rapid recovery after hospitalization, displaying fewer fears, less crying, and less disturbed sleep than children in the control group.

In sum, credible instructions provided in a sympathetic and supportive way that help people avoid attributional errors and that avoid new reasons for anxiety might be more helpful to the complaining patient than blanket reassurances that provide no alternative framework for understanding his symptoms. Reassurance that does not take into account the patient's assessment of the threat that he faces might serve only to mystify him and to undermine his confidence in his physician. The literature contains frequent reports not only of patients with hypochondria who went from one doctor to another but also of repeated cases in which the patient appeared to get gratification in disconfirming the doctor's appraisal. Therapeutic approaches that facilitate the patient's coping efforts may be particularly useful with these difficult patients.

References

1. Gardner, EA: Emotional disorders in medical practice. Ann Intern Med 73:651–653, 1970
2. Gillespie RD: Hypochondria: its definition, nosology and psychopathology. Guys Hosp Rep 8:408–460, 1928
3. Ladee GA: Hypochondriacal Syndromes. Amsterdam, Elsevier Publishing Company, 1966
4. White KL, Williams TF, Greenberg BG: The ecology of medical care. N Engl J Med 265:885–892, 1961
5. United States National Center for Health Statistics. Health Survey Procedure: Concepts, questionnaire development, and definitions in the health interview survey (PHS Publication No 1000, Series 1, No. 2). Washington, DC, Government Printing Office, May, 1964. p 4
6. Mooney HW: Methodology in Two California Health Surveys, San Jose (1952)

and statewide (1954–55). (PHS Monograph No 70) Washington, DC, Government Printing Office, 1963

7. Mechanic D, Newton M: Some problems in the analysis of morbidity data. J Chronic Dis 18:569–580, 1965

8. Woods SM, Natterson J, Silverman J: Medical students' disease: hypochondriasis in medical education. J Med Educ 41:785–790, 1966

9. Hunter RCA, Lohrenz JG, Schwartzman AE: Nosophobia and hypochondriasis in medical students. J Nerv Ment Dis 139:147–152, 1964

10. Schachter S, Singer JE: Cognitive, social, and physiological determinants of emotional state. Psychol Rev 69:379–399, 1962

11. Katzenelbogen S: Hypochondriacal complaints with special reference to personality and environment. Am J Psychiatry 98:815–822, 1942

12. Greenberg HP: Hypochondriasis. Med J Aust 1 (18):673–677, 1960

13. Robins E, Purtell JJ, Cohen ME: "Hysteria" in men: a study of 38 patients so diagnosed and 194 control subjects. N Engl J Med 246:677–685, 1952

14. Kenyon FE: Hypochondriasis: a clinical study. Br J Psychiatry 110:478–488, 1964

15. Srole L., Langner TS, Michael ST, et al: Mental Health in the Metropolis: The Midtown Manhattan study. New York, McGraw-Hill Book Company, 1962

16. Leighton DC, Harding JS, Macklin DB, et al: The Character of Danger: Psychiatric symptoms in selected communities. New York, Basic Books, 1963

17. Brown F: The bodily complaint: a study of hypochondriasis. J Ment Sci 82:295–359, 1936

18. Janis IL: Air War and Emotional Stress: Psychological studies of bombing and civilian defense. New York, McGraw-Hill Book Company, 1951

19. Wolfenstein M: Disaster: A psychological essay. New York, Free Press, 1957

20. Grinker RR, Spiegel JP: Men Under Stress. Philadelphia, Blakiston Publishing Company, 1945

21. Mechanic D: Students Under Stress: A study in the social psychology of adaptation. New York, Free Press, 1962

22. Leventhal H: Findings and theory in the study of fear communications. Adv Exp Soc Psychol 5:119–186, 1970

23. Lazarus RS: Psychological Stress and the Coping Process. New York, McGraw-Hill Book Company, 1966

24. Mechanic, D: The influence of mothers on their children's health attitudes and behavior. Pediatrics 33:444–453, 1964

25. Zborowski M: Cultural components in responses to pain. J Soc Issues 8 (4):16–30, 1952

26. Mechanic, D: Medical Sociology: A selective view. New York, Free Press, 1968

27. Idem: Religion, religiosity, and illness behavior: the special case of the Jews. Hum Organ 22:202–208, 1963

28. Fink R, Shapiro S, Goldensohn SS, et al: The "filter-down" process to psychotherapy in a group practice medical care program. Am J Public Health 59:245–260, 1969

29. Kerckhoff AC, Back KW: The June Bug: A study of hysterical contagion. New York, Appleton-Century-Crofts, 1968

30. Bart PB: Social structure and vocabularies of discomfort: what happened to female hysteria? J Health Soc Behav 9:188–193, 1968

31. Balint M: The Doctor, his Patient and the Illness. New York, International Universities Press, 1957

32. Wolff HG: Headache and Other Head Pain. Second edition. New York, Oxford University Press, 1963
33. Hes JP: Hypochondriacal complaints in Jewish psychiatric patients. Isr Ann Psychiatry 6:134–142, 1968
34. Mechanic D, Volkart EH: Stress, illness behavior, and the sick role. Am Sociol Rev 26:51–58, 1961
35. Mechanic D: Some implications of illness behavior for medical sampling. N Engl J Med 269:244–247, 1963
36. Mechanic D, Jackson D: Stress, Illness Behavior, and the Use of General Practitoner Services: A study of British women (mimeographed). Madison, Department of Sociology, University of Wisconsin
37. Kadushin C: Individual decisions to undertake psychotherapy. Adm Sci Q 3:379–411, 1958
38. Beecher HK: Measurement of Subjective Responses: quantitative effects of drugs. New York, Oxford University Press, 1959
39. Lambert WE, Libman E, Poser EG: The effect of increased salience of a membership group on pain tolerance. J Pers 28:350–357, 1960
40. Ross L, Rodin J, Zimbardo PG: Toward an attribution therapy: the reduction of fear through induced cognitive-emotional misattribution. J Pers Soc Psychol 12:279–288, 1969
41. Blitz B, Dinnerstein AJ: Role of attentional focus in pain perception: manipulation of response to noxious stimulation by instructions. J Abnorm Psychol 77:42–45, 1971
42. Walters A: Psychogenic regional pain alias hysterical pain. Brain 84:1–18, 1961
43. Imboden JB, Canter A, Cluff LE, et al: Brucellosis. III. Psychologic aspects of delayed convalescence. Arch Intern Med 103:406–414, 1959
44. Imboden JB, Canter A, Cluff L: Symptomatic recovery from medical disorders: influence of psychological factors. JAMA 178:1182–1184, 1961
45. Zola IK: Problems of communication, diagnosis, and patient care: the interplay of patient, physician and clinic organization. J Med Educ 38:829–838, 1963
46. Brodman K, Mittelmann B, Wechsler D, et al: The relation of personality disturbances to duration of convalescence from acute respiratory infections. Psychosom Med 9:37–44, 1947
47. Rickels K, Downing RW: Drug- and placebo-treated neurotic outpatients: pretreatment levels of manifest anxiety, clinical improvement, and side reactions. Arch Gen Psychiatry 16:369–372, 1967
48. Rickels K, Lipman R, Raab E: Previous medication, duration of illness and placebo response. J Nerv Ment Dis 142:548–554, 1966
49. Storms MD, Nisbett RE: Insomnia and the attribution process. J Pers Soc Psychol 16:319–328, 1970
50. Egbert LD, Battit GE, Welch CE, et al: Reduction of postoperative pain by encouragement and instruction of patients: a study of doctor-patient rapport. N Engl J Med 270:825–827, 1964
51. Skipper JK Jr, Leonard RC: Children, stress, and hospitalization: a field experiment, J. Health Soc Behav 9:275–287, 1968

8

Patient Behavior and the Organization of
Medical Care

Throughout most of the history of medicine, physicians could do little to prevent disease or to intervene effectively in its progress. But people sought the assistance of physicians, healers, and shamans to relieve their sense of subjective distress and uncertainty. Seeking care was in part a symbol of continuing hope, in part an expression of a desire to alleviate pain and restore functional capacity. These basic human needs persist today as well, perhaps overshadowed by the scientific development and technical elaboration of medical activities, but have a profound effect on the perception and response to medical services.

It is trite to observe that persons live in families and communities and that these social contexts shape their perceptions and behavior. Nevertheless it is true that how people come to identify problems, why they become concerned about them, and how and when they seek assistance are influenced by their social context as much as they are by objective symptoms or the character of the medical care system; and their reactions to treatment, their willingness to return to the physician, and cooperation in following medical advice are all affected by the extent to which the medical context conforms or clashes with social and cultural expectations.

The medical practitioner, by virtue of his activities, is in a position from which it is difficult to obtain an unbiased view of the social behavior systems affecting the occurrence of illness and the responses to it. The persons he ordinarily sees are those who have selected themselves for care, and the practitioner has little basis for an accurate construction of the populations from which the patients were selected, or how they are different from those who did not seek care. Even a cursory examination of the potential population at risk demonstrates considerable overlap in presenting symptoms between patients who seek care and symptoms reported by others in the population who do not choose to consult a physician.

Using relatively conservative estimates of the occurrence of physical symptoms in the population—that is, symptom reports based on an action criterion such as taking bed rest or medication—it is apparent that a large proportion of the population, approximately three quarters, have symptoms in any given month comparable to those that physicians see every day.[1] Approximately only one in three of these patients will seek a consultation with a physician. These estimates are based largely on acute and chronic physical illness and do not consider the wide range of psychiatric morbidity in the population. Estimates of such morbidity are difficult to provide since they vary so substantially from one study to another depending on the criterion used.[2] Obviously, if the criterion is too loose, the category becomes too inclusive. Various studies suggest that an estimate that from 5 to 10 percent of the population have serious psychiatric problems requiring care—such as depression, alcoholism, and the like—would be conservative.[3] Some epidemiological studies have reported that as many as 60 percent of the population suffer from psychiatric impairment.

To understand the process of medical care, it is essential to understand why some patients decide to seek care and others do not, why care seeking is initiated at particular points in time, and how the needs of patients and their motivations for medical care interact with the organization of the delivery system.

Differences in response to symptoms are dependent on the manner in which problems become manifest and their severity, on the social and cultural background and experience of the persons involved, and on the immediate contingencies of patients' life situations.[4] But before elaborating on each of these points, it is useful to examine what people mean by health, and how it relates to medical conceptions.

Although persons in Western nations have a fairly sophisticated view of health and illness, it is quite different from the professional viewpoint of physicians. Medicine as a science has developed by making abstract distinctions and classifications that have been incorporated in the way in which physicians define and treat patients. Patients react to illness more experientially and in a fashion that does not distinguish between feeling states and specific symptoms. Health is a state of perception and experience, and not the absence of one or another disease entity. Thus, when the correlates of persons' perceptions of their physical health are examined, psychological distress is a major predictor of how they see themselves.

Since reactions to illness are largely experiential, it is not surprising that persons who have symptoms are more likely to define them as worthy of care when such symptoms disrupt their ability to function and interfere in some fashion with their life activities. Investigators have consistently observed that illness is most salient when it is disruptive to usual functions, activities, and routines.[5] However, the seriousness of symptoms from a medical perspective may or may not be related to their salience or disruptiveness. Patients are also more likely to define symptoms as worthy of care when bodily indications are unfamiliar and frightening and when the person lacks an interpretation that allows "normalization" of the symptom. Some symptoms are much more easily normalized than others; chest pains might be attributed to indigestion, muscle ache to physical activity, or headaches to tension and stress.

How people react to symptoms is also related to their prior learning and experience and to the cultural and social definitions of the groups within which they live. Some years ago I characterized this concern as the study of illness behavior, and a fair amount of information on such reactions has accumulated in the last decade. Individuals as part of their social development acquire various attitudes and behaviors that are in part characteristic of their social contexts. Some groups encourage the expression of distress, while others expect stoicism and denial. Some cultural contexts provide a detailed psychological vocabulary to conceptualize and describe personal problems, while others communicate disapproval of any such suggestions.[6] These norms differ not only among social and ethnic groups but also may vary for men and women, children and adults. Such norms—and experience in reference to them—come to have an important effect on how persons define their difficulties in functioning and how they adapt to life problems.

Going to a doctor is only one of many possible responses for persons suffering pain and distress or disruption in life activities. In some of our studies we have attempted to measure in a rather crude way the varying propensity of persons to go to a doctor when they face illness. In some subgroups persons learn to seek out physicians readily when they have a problem, to have faith in doctors, and to have little skepticism about the value of medical care. In other contexts, learning experiences lead to delay in seeking medical care, denial of symptoms, and little trust in doctors. These propensities are not unfixed or unchanging, but frequently interact with the organization and typical response of the health care system and other factors in the individual's environment.

Various studies indicate that life difficulties and psychological distress are frequently present among persons seeking medical care.[7] Such stressful life situations have been alleged to contribute to the occurrence of illness, and this indeed may be the case.[8] But as Balint[9] has maintained, life difficulties and psychological distress frequently trigger the use of physician services, although some physical symptom might be presented as a justification for coming to see the doctor. Thus the high rate of psychological distress among patients seen may result either because such distress contributes to symptoms and illness, contributes to illness behavior and help seeking, or both. Our research suggests that psychological distress appears to have a larger influence among patients with high readiness to use physician services. Among patients with less readiness and greater skepticism of medical care, psychological distress may result in other forms of coping.

There are limits within which discretion in help seeking operates. When symptoms are sufficiently acute and severe, the impact of definitional processes is limited. But when symptoms occur less dramatically, in a milder form, and have limited impact on functioning, such social processes may be crucial. Much of ambulatory care falls within this latter categorization, and thus social definitions and response have an important impact on the content and process of primary care.

In part, patients who seek medical care as a result of life difficulties and high readiness to depend on physicians may present their problems in a variety of ways, and underlying problems are frequently identified only with difficulty. Some patients, of course, have a highly developed psychosocial vocabulary and present their problems to the doctor in psychosomatic and psychosocial frames of reference. They may complain of family conflict, depression, difficulties on the job, or whatever. Studies indicate that patients with such constructions of their complaints tend to be more urban, more educated, and tend to come from backgrounds encouraging a psychological vocabulary—such as among Jewish populations. A second type of patient, however, chronically complains of diffuse physical symptoms that are characteristic of both psychological and physical disorder: loss of appetite, difficulty sleeping, fatigue, aches and pains, and so on. Such patients are more likely to be of rural origins, to have less education, and to come from cultural backgrounds that discourage the open expression of emotions and complaints. Various data suggest that these patients subject themselves to considerable diagnostic work and to a high prevalence of surgical procedures. Other types of presentations fall between these two extreme types. A common complaint by patients is "nerves," a category between a physical and psychological presentation. Patients describing their problem as one of "nerves" frequently resist any interpretation that directly implicates factors in their immediate life situations, but seem to recognize their problems as somewhat different than more conventional physical disorders. Finally, many patients presenting self-limited acute complaints of mild or moderate severity may have come to the doctor as much because of life difficulties as of the symptom presented. But, then again, the physician does not really know, and that contributes enormously to the difficulty of his task. Let us now consider how this all appears from the physician's perspective.

Physician Responses to Patient Complaints

The capacity of the doctor to cope effectively with the types of problems characteristic of primary medical care depends not only on his personality, attitudinal orientations, and prior preparation but also on the practice pressures and incentives he faces and the manner in which care is organized. The physician must manage not only his patients but also his time so as to complete the day's work and be reasonably responsive to his patients in the aggregate. How he does this will depend on both the organization of his practice and incentives implicit in how he is paid.

The discussion that follows must be somewhat exploratory since there is very limited research on how practice structures affect the physician's behavior. I, therefore, must depend substantially on my own inquiries that have certain limitations. Most serious of these limitations is that the studies that I will report are cross-sectional and nonexperimental in character and depend exclusively on what the physician reports about himself and his practice. When one observes an association in nonexperimental, cross-sectional studies between a mode of practice and other behavior, it is impossible to precisely determine to what extent the outcome is attributable to organizational effects from the degree to which certain persons with particular behavioral orientations select certain modes of practice. Also, without independent observations, self-reports of physicians concerning their own work must be viewed with a certain skepticism. Wherever possible, I seek data from other studies that either strengthen or contradict my conclusions, but I emphasize that the types of investigations I discuss cannot prove the contentions I will put forth.

When I first became interested in general medical practice in England and Wales in the early 1960s, I was impressed by the frequency with which practitioners complained of the triviality and inappropriateness of medical consultations. As I inquired into the issue I became more puzzled because the usual interpretations of the reasons for such complaints appeared to be inconsistent with existing information. Although there was a tendency to explain such attributions of triviality by the fact that the National Health Service was free—and thus the argument that the absence of economic barriers led to exploitation of the doctor—the available data on practitioner utilization could not sustain this contention. Average medical utilization was not substantially higher in England than in the United States, nor was it likely that differences in utilization or patients' behavior from one practitioner to another could account for their widely varying attributions of triviality. Also, it appeared that doctors with larger panels complained more vigorously of trivial patients; yet existing data suggested that the patients of such doctors had lower average per capita utilization of medical services than patients of doctors with smaller panels. I came to the same conclusion as Ann Cartwright,[10] who was also working on similar issues at the time, that the attributions of triviality told us more about the doctor and his practice than about the objective characteristics of his patients or the nature of their problems.

When we examine the reports of official bodies—such as the Gillie Committee[11] or the Royal Commission on Medical Education[12]—we find that the dissatisfaction of physicians and their frustrations are explained by such factors as a lack of hospital attachment, the absence of group practice or adequate ancillary help, or the unsatisfactory educational preparation of the general practitioner. When we studied a national sample of general practitioners in 1965–1966, we could find little evidence in support of any of these arguments except that doctors with training in psychiatry and behavioral science seemed somewhat more content.[13] We cannot determine whether this is attributable to the training or to the types of people who select to have such training. I should emphasize that our sample of 800 general practitioners did not provide many who were working in modern practice structures, containing the advantages usually attributed to group or health center practice or to the effective use of paraprofessional manpower. Thus, it is conceivable that the implementation of the suggestions of these official committees could have a real effect. But within the prevalent variations then existing, I am frankly skeptical.

In the study of English general practitioners a large number of variables was examined. Most variables describing the doctor's background or modes of practice had little effect on how he viewed his patients or his own satisfactions and dissatisfactions. Only one type of factor appeared to matter very much—patient demand. The more patients the doctor saw, the more likely he was to describe them as trivial and inappropriate. The influence of patient demand was pronounced even when controlling many other variables simultaneously.

Such an association is, of course, open to a variety of interpretations. We were able to exclude some of these since we had collected a great deal of data on various facets of the doctor's practice. One could not account for the differences on the basis of geographic area or the doctors' descriptions of the social class characteristics of their patients. Nor is it likely that the different perceptions of triviality reflect real differences in the distribution of morbidity or help seeking in varying doctors' panels, although this issue deserves more study. I, thus, came to the following *post hoc* interpretation of these findings.

English general practitioners, paid on a weighted capitation basis, develop some concept of how much time they ought to devote to their practices. Although they may adjust to varying patient demands in their practice, they do this within some concept of what constitutes a reasonable workweek. They then establish fixed surgery hours within which they accommodate the patients who wish to see them. Doctors who have larger panels and who schedule more limited surgery hours relative to patient demand must practice an assembly-line medicine that basically involves symptomatic treatment. As patient demand grows, the doctor must practice in a more hurried way to get through the daily queue. The doctor, of course, can cope by increasing his surgery hours substantially, but a capitation system of payment provides no incentive for him doing so. Obviously, some do so because of their own compulsiveness or sense of obligation, but our concern here is with the average tendencies and not the exceptions.

The general practitioner sees many patients with psychosocial problems who suffer from significant psychological distress, and this has been well documented by the studies of general practice carried out by Michael Shepherd and his group.[14] Such patients may present common physical complaints to justify their consultations, but such visits may be motivated by underlying distress. These patients are difficult to care for under the best of circumstances, but under conditions that prevail in the busiest surgeries the doctor has little time to talk with the patient and explore in any detail the nature of his concerns.

The doctor, in treating the patient symptomatically, is aware of his failures to explore the patient's problem and feels frustrated by his manner of practice. The attribution of triviality is probably a reflection of this feeling, and, indeed, we find that doctors who report that a large proportion of their patients are trivial also report that they frequently do not have time to do an adequate examination and to do what is necessary for the patient. They also report more frequently than other doctors that they more commonly issue prescriptions without seeing the patient and give patients certificates although unconvinced that the patient is too sick for work.[15] In short, I am suggesting that British general practitioners define patients as trivial because the nature of their practice induces them to treat patient complaints as if they are trivial.

We anticipated that fee-for-service arrangements would create different incentives for the doctor's behavior; thus, we carried out a similar investigation of a national sample of 1,500 American general practitioners, internists, pediatricians, and obstetricians.[16] Although perceptions of triviality are not uncommon in the American context, such reports are much less frequent than in British practice. In general, American doctors see far fewer patients, and expectations require that they give the patient more time than in typical British practice. We anticipated that, in fee-for-service practice, doctors would be subject to a larger extent to what Freidson has called "client control" and, thus, would anticipate that their patients expect the doctor to spend a reasonable amount of time with them. Because of the fee-for-service incentive, we anticipated that doctors would be more likely to respond to such patient expectations by increasing office hours in order to see patients. Indeed, this is what we and others find. Doctors in fee-for-service practice, who face large patient demand, work very long hours.[17] Unlike the British practitioners, the doctor is rewarded for every additional patient he sees. Consistent with this is the finding that when physicians move from a fee-for-service to a salaried structure, as occurred in Canada, they report a decrease in hours worked.[18]

In the American context, we anticipated that prepaid physicians in large prepaid group practices would be exposed to incentives very much like those characteristic of English general practice. Although our sample of doctors in prepaid groups was very limited within the context of our national sample, our fragmentary data suggested that they responded very much like the English general practitioners and that they were much more likely to attribute triviality or inappropriateness to the patients they see.[19]

This finding was sufficiently provocative so that we selected still another national sample of physicians who practiced in prepaid groups. For reasons that I would not go into here, this sample includes only general practitioners and pediatricians. The analysis of these data is still incomplete, but they suggest a complex and differentiated response depending on the practice conditions prevailing. Consistent with our previous survey of American physicians, general practitioners and pediatricians in prepaid group practice are more than three times as likely as nongroup fee-for-service practitioners to indicate that 50 percent or more of their patients are trivial or inappropriate (Table 8.1). While only 9 percent of nongroup general practitioners report this many patients as trivial, 32 percent of general practitioners in prepaid practice give such a report. The comparable figures for pediatricians are 9 percent and 29 percent. I should note that the proportion of American general practitioners and pediatricians in prepaid practice reporting 50 percent or more of their patients as trivial is higher than the 24 percent of British general practitioners who give such reports.

One possibility, of course, is that prepaid patients exploit medical care in the absence of economic barriers, and perceptions of triviality reflect such abuse. We have carefully examined existing data involving studies of

TABLE 8.1
Reports Concerning Trivial Consultations in Varying Practice Settings

	Percent Reporting 50% or More Patients Are Trivial	Percent Reporting 10% or Less Patients Are Trivial
British general practitioners (N = 772)	24	12
All nongroup American primary care physicians[a] (N = 1148)	7	36
All group American primary care physicians[b] (N = 310)	10	36
Nongroup American general practitioners (N = 604)	9	33
Group American general practitioners (N = 113)	13	27
Nongroup American pediatricians (N = 136)	9	31
Group American pediatricians (N = 43)	9	33
Prepaid American general practitioners[b] (N = 108)	32	7
Prepaid American pediatricians[b] (N = 154)	29	14

[a]Includes general practitioners, pediatricians, internists, and obstetricians.
[b]Includes physicians in practices involving 50 percent or more prepaid practice activity.

prepaid practice and utilization data reported by the large prepaids, such as Health Insurance Plan and Kaiser-Portland. In some cases, average utilization in prepaid practice is a little higher than in other forms of practice; in some cases, there are no clear differences; and in still other cases there is even evidence of lower rates of utilization than in the population at large.[20] This should not be surprising in that we know that there are many noneconomic barriers that control rates of utilization: the resources made available, distance to the outpatient facility, difficulty in making an appointment, waiting time, and the responsiveness of care once one arrives.

On the basis of our two earlier surveys, we suspected that physicians in prepaid contexts viewed themselves as working on a contractual basis. They receive a fixed salary for a defined period of work, and unlike fee-for-service physicians, there are few existing incentives to substantially increase the amount of time they spend seeing patients. Thus we suspected that when prepaid practices faced large patient demands, they scheduled extra patients within the physicians' defined hours of work rather than have the physicians work longer hours. This would result in a more assembly-line practice, one that is less responsive to the patient as a person. Studies of consumers of prepaid practice also report that they are more likely than in fee-for-service practice to feel that practitioners are less responsive to their needs and seem less interested in them, [21,22] and this is consistent with the overall agrument.

When we more closely examined the specific components of the physicians' satisfactions and dissatisfactions in our large American sample, we found support for this interpretation. Fee-for-service physicians have longer workweeks than prepaid physicians and complain the most of their long hours of work and lack of leisure time. In contrast, prepaid group practitioners are more satisfied with their overall workweek, but they are more dissatisfied with the amount of time for each patient.

Our sample of general practitioners and pediatricians in prepaid group practice provided a further opportunity to examine factors affecting the perceptions and attributions of physicians working on other than fee-for-service arrangements. As we anticipated, physicians in prepaid practice are much more likely to have a shorter workweek, although they spend more of their total working time in direct patient care. Doctors in prepaid practice, in contrast to both other group and nongroup practitioners, are more satisfied with the total time their medical practice requires and with the leisure time available to them. Although prepaid group general practitioners were most likely to be dissatisfied with the time available for each patient, this expected relationship was not obtained for the prepaid group pediatricians. Unexpectedly, we found the opposite to be the case: The nongroup pediatricians were most dissatisfied with having adequate time for each patient. This finding required a more detailed examination of the practice characteristics of nongroup and prepaid group pediatricians.

Our data conform with the typical picture of the highly harassed nongroup pediatrician. In comparison to the prepaid group pediatricians, nongroup pediatricians saw many more patients, worked many more hours, and took on a wider range of functions and responsibilities. For example, on the previous day, 43 percent of nongroup pediatricians saw 33 or more patients in contrast to 18 percent of prepaid group pediatricians who saw this many. More than half of the nongroup pediatricians reported seeing this many patients on a typical busy day, but only 34 percent of prepaid group pediatricians gave a comparable report. While 31 percent of nongroup pediatricians reported that they saw more patients than reasonable, only 13 percent of group prepaid pediatricians gave a similar report. Furthermore, nongroup pediatricians reported spending more time on the phone, on hospital rounds, on administrative work, and the like. They made more house calls and spent more time managing their practice. In contrast, although prepaid group general practitioners had a much shorter workweek than nongroup practitioners, they saw a large number of patients when they worked. Two fifths of the prepaid group general practitioners saw 33 or more patients on the previous day, and 37 percent reported that they had responsibility for more patients than was reasonable.

Because of the different practice demands faced by prepaid group general practitioners and pediatricians, we pursued the analysis separately for each group. While such reports as having responsibility for too many patients were associated with reported trivial consultations among prepaid general practitioners, they were not very useful as predictors among prepaid group pediatricians who faced a much smaller patient load. We thus examined all of our samples of physicians to establish those findings that were consistently associated with attributions of triviality across all samples. As a consequence, we ignored many strong findings that appeared in some samples but not in others. For example, among prepaid group general practitioners, the correlation between the doctors' disagrement that they have a "responsibility to advise and care for the psychological problems of patients" and the proportion of patients perceived as trivial is 0.34; among prepaid group pediatricians it is 0.14; and in the overall sample of American primary care physicians it is only 0.07. By the criterion stated above, the association between these two variables would not be regarded as stable, but it is probably suggestive of the true complexity of the phenomenon at issue. I suspect that the relationship between perceived responsibility for psychological problems and attributions of triviality is only strong when the physician is paid on a capitation basis and when he has more patients than he can reasonably cope with. At present we are pursuing these ideas in a multi-variate analysis.

In examining those correlations consistent throughout all samples, we find that attributions of triviality are associated with concern about people bringing less serious disorders to doctors and more readily seeking help for problems in their family lives and with less overall satisfaction. We also find that attributions of triviality are consistently higher among physicians who report that they are dissatisfied with the amount of time they have for each patient and among those who report seeing more patients on a busy day. We suspect that attributions of triviality reflect the reactions of a technically inclined physician burdened by a heavy patient load and with few incentives to be responsive to the psychological and social concerns that are associated with many patient consultations.

These findings reinforce our understanding that each type of practice organization has its own distinctive advantages and disadvantages. There is a great deal of data suggesting that a fee-for-service system, in the absence of other controls, promotes incentives for unnecessary and perhaps dangerous work and increases the rate of discretionary surgery.[23] Physicians in this type of practice frequently work themselves to exhaustion, taking insufficient time for continuing education and leisure. The direct dependence on the patient's satisfaction, however, may produce a more responsive attitude and one that communicates greater interest in and concern for the patient. This may be reflected in a greater willingness on the part of the physician to answer the patient's inquiries, to talk with him, and to have an interest in his viewpoint.

In prepaid group practice the physician is less attuned to his patient, and as Freidson[24] has suggested, colleague control is more prevalent. This may be conducive to a high quality of technical medical care and an avoidance of unnecessary treatment, but it also may be conducive to a certain inflexibility and lack of responsiveness that may not be consistent with a high level of primary care. The point is not to engage in mindless polemics about the value of one or another system of organization, but to seek models of care that maximize the advantages and minimize the costs of each. In talking about new models of primary medical care, we must be continually aware of the human problems of medical care and the factors that bring patients to physicians in the first place.[25]

A certain level of morale is necessary for decent performance, and we should bolster physician morale as much as possible to the extent that it does not undermine other functions. I believe that we must combine the advantages of prepaid group practice with new incentives for physicians who work within such practice contexts. The most important goal of such incentives would be to make the physician more responsive and interested in the types of problems typical of ambulatory care. Since such responsiveness is closely associated with the number of patients the physician is responsible for and the types of problems they have, we cannot neglect the issue of the amount and types of patient demand, the effective use of ancillary assistance, and the implementation of new paraprofessionals as a way of dealing more effectively with some of the problems discussed.

Consideration of Alternative Innovations in Primary Medical Care

In discussing patient motivation in seeking medical care, I maintained that psychological concerns were of great importance. From a practical point of view we might distinguish services for such patients in terms of the complexity of their needs. Conservative estimates suggest that approximately 5 to 10 percent of patient populations have formal psychiatric difficulties and that of these approximately 5 percent are acutely psychotic. Some proportion of this group is clearly beyond the capabilities and experience of the typical primary care physician and requires referral. The remainder of this group is probably manageable within primary medical care with supportive specialty assistance for the primary physician. Beyond this group of formal disorders are others that require time and attention but no complicated regimen. Then there are many chronic patients with considerable psychological and psychosocial problems who could be served quite effectively on a continuing basis by nurse-practitioners supported by the primary care physician.[26]

There is now increasing evidence that providing psychiatric assistance to chronically complaining patients is related to an overall reduction in medical and hospital utilization.[27] However, since these studies tend to be nonexperimental, it is difficult to project whether the same outcomes can be achieved among chronic complainers who now resist psychiatric care or a psychiatric interpretation of their problem.[28] Such patients are probably better managed by the primary care physician. It is important to also note that the utilization reduction reported in these studies mainly characterizes patients with mild and moderate disorders. The seriously disturbed psychiatric patients do not appear to reduce overall medical utilization despite the provision of psychiatric care.

Primary care physicians treat the vast majority of patients with psychiatric disorders. Only a relatively small proportion is referred, or refer themselves, to psychiatric facilities. This process of pathways into psychiatric care has been extensively studied, and for the less extreme disorders it is clear that social and cultural characteristics are important in determining the use of psychiatric referral.[29] Patients more willing to accept psychiatric referral are better educated, more cosmopolitan, and are more likely to associate with others who have used or are receptive to psychiatric services. Also, such receptivity is more common in urban areas, among particular ethnic groups such as Jews, and among persons with lower religiosity.

No matter how good psychiatric services are—and they are far from optimal—much of the responsibility will continue to reside with the primary care physician. Many primary care physicians have negative attitudes toward both psychiatry and psychiatric patients, and rates of recognition and referral of psychiatric patients fluctuate widely from one practitioner to another.[30] But regardless of the attitude of physicians, the management of patients with psychiatric and psychosocial difficulties can be exceedingly difficult. Some probably need no more than a professional who expresses an interest in their problems and who is willing to listen to them, but the patient with diffuse physical complaints who may indeed have a serious physical condition poses a much more difficult problem.

Physicians, of course, have an obligation to satisfy themselves that the complaints have no basis in detectable organic disease, but if they are not to exaggerate such physical detection processes, they must also be attentive to patients' psychological states and provide opportunities for relevant psychological and social information to become salient. Many complaining patients are significantly depressed and anxious, but do not feel free to discuss these feelings unless the physician provides an appropriate opening.

There is growing evidence that indicates that dealing with many psychosocial problems requires more than social support and encouragement that contributes to the reduction of feelings of anxiety and distress.[31] In many circumstances patients require specific instructions that assist them in dealing with their life circumstances. To be effective, such instructions must be relevant to their problem and consistent with the patient's experiences, and they also must be psychologically and culturally credible. The growing utility of behavior modification approaches offers some promise for the practitioner dealing with problems of child care, obesity, alcohol abuse, and the like. In many areas of behavior, it is not clear what directions for behavior change are credible, but it is valuable for the practitioner to keep in mind not only the needs of the patient to maintain greater psychological comfort but also the necessary instructions and skills required for the patient to cope with his or her life situation.

I emphasize the dimension of credibility since every practitioner knows that there is a substantial difference between recognizing a patient's level of psychological distress and obtaining the acceptance of the patient that this is part of the problem. I also noted that there are many persons who resist psychological attributions to their distress because of prior cultural upbringing and existing social norms in their important primary groups. The physician who forces a definition on a patient that the patient is unprepared to accept achieves little and may undermine whatever source of help he can be. He must work patiently and subtly within the patient's frame of reference if he is to achieve desired results.

If, indeed, this is part of the responsibility of primary care physicians, it is not difficult to understand why a technically efficient and operationally hurried practice may not be conducive to its fulfillment. The realities of care require certain trade-offs between optimally responsive care and the need to meet demands for access to the physician, but we would do well to recognize what it is that is sacrificed and attempt to develop appropriate models of care that are better attuned to the forces that create concern in the population and that bring patients into medical care.

Implications for the Resolution of Conflicts

The problem in meeting patient expectations is inherent in the different conceptions of physician and patient and in the conflict between giving patients more comprehensive care in contrast to seeing more patients. To the extent that physicians take a broad view of their responsibilities, and devote time to exploring life situations and providing support and advice, curtailment of patient load becomes mandatory. When resources are limited, however, those without adequate access to care might not experience such modifications as beneficial.

It should be apparent that patients have diverse needs and orientations, and no simple uniform assumptions will allow physicians to proceed effectively. If the physician is to respond to the patient as an individual, he must have some acquaintance with him and be sensitive to changing needs, and this requires time and continuity. Physicians, of course, complain that they lack the time and, in any case, it is not clear to them that such investments yield much in the way of tangible benefits. Thus physicians focus on identifying and treating recognizable disease states that are relatively clear-cut, subject to routinization, and are consistent with the models of behavior with which the physician has learned to feel comfortable.

The more specialized approach to the patient has other consequences as well. In focusing on the search for disease, which is largely a technical activity, the physician can proceed in a manner less dependent on the patient or on his cooperation and involvement. Thus, the physician can deal with the patient as an object with little attention to the patient's wishes or consent. He proceeds independently, making decisions on the tests to order, the procedures to use, and the expenses involved. Even with such major decisions as hospitalization, length of stay, and the use of discretionary procedures, the involvement of the patient is usually limited to providing nominal or legal consent. The organization of medical activity generally is one that leaves the patient with the impression of being worked on and is hardly conducive to maximize the play of the patient's values and choices against those characterizing the predominant medical approach.

While in ambulatory settings the pressures of time and the limited scope of the physician's approach result in constraints on patient expression and choice, such constraints are greatly exacerbated by the elaboration of conflicting interests in multipurpose institutions such as teaching hospitals and medical centers.[32] In such contexts there is an elaboration of potential conflicts of interest between patients' wishes and the constellation of pressures on the physician from patient load, service needs, research, and teaching. As these institutional forms have grown and as new programs have emerged, such conflicts are actually built in as a way of coping with particular problems. Thus, a health maintenance organization (HMO) may provide economic incentives for the physician to cut down patient utilization of services, a teaching hospital may give awards to the house officers who achieve the greatest participation of patients in research work[33] or who get the most autopsy permissions,[34] and patients may be kept in the hospital to protect and enhance the vitality of a developing unit that requires a minimum patient load to ensure its continued financing.

The existing pressures toward specialization and bureaucratization of medical work—and the emphasis on efficiency and productivity—make it difficult to reorder priorities in a way that ensures patient care that is responsive to them as persons rather than as objects, that maximizes opportunities for expression and choice, and that provides occasions for participation and instruction in relationships with professionals. But if one measures the success of medical care by its effective implementation rather than by the number of consultations and number of procedures performed, then what now appears inefficient and wasteful may turn out not to be as costly as alleged. Current medical practice is characterized by frequent disruptions in communication, in unsatisfactory relationships between patients and physicians and in frequent failure to conform with medical advice.[35] Care that is responsive to patient perceptions and expectations, that provides the patient an opportunity to be heard, and that instructs the patient in a fashion consistent with knowledge of life situations and problems may result in greater cooperation and implementation of medical care.

In conclusion, I do not want to exaggerate what we know about managing human problems in the context of medical care. Serious research in this relatively neglected area is of high priority. From the perspective of human values, however, medicine has a social role that far transcends the technical procedures that doctors perform. To deny these needs and motivations is to debase the practice of medicine and its traditions. In social life symbols are of immense importance, and the character of medical activities and their scope help define those aspects of man that we value.

I also would not want to minimize the practical issues. The implementation of comprehensive medicine depends on a more adequate distribution of medical manpower, better models for organizing health care tasks between physicians and among health workers generally, and the development of new educational settings in which the larger problems of medical practice are given attention as a major priority in the work of faculty and the training of students. This is not possible without fundamental changes in medical education and medical practice, and in the reward structures that determine not what people say but how they behave.

References

1. White KL, Williams TF, Greenberg GB: The ecology of medical care. N Engl J Med 265:885–892, 1961.
2. Dohrenwend B, Dohrenwend B: Social Status and Psychological Disorder. New York, Wiley Interscience, 1969.
3. Gardner E: Emotional disorders in medical practice. Ann Intern Med 73:651–652, 1970.
4. Mechanic D: Public Expectations and Health Care. New York, Wiley Interscience, 1972, pp. 203–222.
5. Mechanic D: Medical Sociology. New York, Free Press, 1968, pp. 145–146.
6. Mechanic D: Social psychologic factors affecting the presentation of bodily complaints. N Engl J Med 286:1132–1139, 1972.
7. Shepherd M: Psychiatric Illness in General Practice. London, Oxford University Press, 1966.
8. Hinkle LE, Jr: The effect of exposure to culture change, social change, and changes in interpersonal relationships upon health. Presented at the Conference on Stressful Life Events, University Center of the City of New York, June 1973.
9. Balint M: The Doctor, His Patient and the Illness. New York, International Universities Press, 1957.
10. Cartwright A: Patients and Their Doctors: A Study of General Practice. London, Routledge, 1967.
11. Great Britain Ministry of Health: The Field of Work of the Family Doctor. London, Her Majesty's Stationery Office, 1963.
12. Royal Commission on Medical Education, 1965–68 Report. London, Her Majesty's Stationery Office, 1968 (Cmnd 3569).

13. Mechanic D: Correlates of frustration among British general practitioners. J. Health Soc Behav 11:87–104, 1970.
14. Shepherd M: *op. cit.*
15. Mechanic D: Correlates of frustration among British general practitioners. *op. cit.*
16. Mechanic D: General medical practice: some comparisons between the work of primary care physicians in the United States and England and Wales. Med Care 10:402–420, 1972.
17. *Ibid.*
18. Enterline PE, et al: Effect of "free" medical care on medical practice—the Quebec experience. N Engl J Med 288:1152–1155, 1973.
19. Mechanic D: Physician satisfaction in varying settings. Paper presented at the NCHSRD Manpower Conference, Chicago, Illinois, 1971.
20. Health Insurance Plan of New York: H.I.P. Statistical Report: 1968–1969. New York, Division of Research and Statistics, 1970; Saward E, et al.: Documentation of twenty years of operation and growth of a prepaid group practice plan. Med Care 6:239–244, 1968; Columbia School of Public Health and Administrative Medicine: Family Medical Care under Three Types of Health Insurance. New York, Foundation on Employee Health, Medical Care and Welfare, Inc., 1962; Committee for the Special Research Project in the Health Insurance Plan of New York: Health and Medical Care in New York City. Cambridge, Harvard University Press, 1957; Darsky BJ, et al: Comprehensive Medical Services under Voluntary Health Insurance. Cambridge, Harvard University Press, 1958; Anderson OW, Sheatsley PB: Comprehensive Medical Insurance: A Study of Costs, Use and Attitudes under Two Plans, New York, Health Information Foundation Research Ser No 9, 1959.
21. Freidson E: Patients' Views of Medical Practice. New York, Russell Sage Foundation, 1961.
22. Donabedian A: A review of some experiences with prepaid group practice. Bureau of Public Health Economics Research Ser No 12. Ann Arbor, School of Public Health, University of Michigan, 1965.
23. Roemer MI: On paying the doctor and the implications of different methods. J Health Human Behav 3:4–14, 1962; U.S. Department of Health, Education, and Welfare: Toward a Comprehensive Health Policy for the 1970s: A White Paper. Washington, D.C., Government Printing Office, 1971.
24. Freidson E: Profession of Medicine. New York, Dodd, Mead, 1970.
25. Mechanic D: Public Expectations and Health Care. *op. cit.,* pp. 67–79.
26. Lewis CE, Resnik BA: Nurse clinics and progressive ambulatory patient care. N Engl J Med 277:1236–1241, 1967.
27. Follette W, Cummings NA: Psychiatric services and medical utilization in a prepaid health plan setting. Med Care 5:25–35, 1967; Goldberg ID, et al: Effect of a short-term outpatient psychiatric therapy benefit on the utilization of medical services in a prepaid group practice medical program. Med Care 8:419–428, 1970.
28. Follette W, Cummings NA: Psychiatric services and medical utilization in a prepaid health care setting. Part II. Med Care 6:31–41, 1968.
29. Kadushin C: Why People Go to Psychiatrists. New York, Atherton, 1969.
30. Shepherd M: *op. cit.*
31. Leventhal H: Findings and theory in the study of fear communications. Adv Exp Soc Psychol 5:119–186, 1970; Egbert LD, et al.: Reduction of postopera-

tive pain by encouragement and instruction of patients: a study of doctor–patient rapport. N Engl J Med 270:825–827, 1964.

32. Duff RS, Hollingshead AB: Sickness and Society. New York, Harpers, 1968; Cartwright A: Human Relations and Hospital Care. Boston, Routledge and Kegan Paul, 1964.
33. Miller S: Prescription for Leadership: Training for the Medical Elite. Chicago, Aldine, 1970.
34. Duff RS, Hollingshead AB: *op. cit.*
35. Ley P, Spelman MS: Communicating with the Patient. London, Trinity Press, 1967.

Part III
RESEARCH ISSUES AND APPROACHES

9

Correlates of Physician Utilization: Why Do Major Multivariate Studies of Physician Utilization Find Trivial Psychosocial and Organizational Effects?

There appears to be a major contradiction in the literature in medical sociology on the determinants of physician utilization. On the one hand, there is an extensive literature dealing with sociocultural, organizational, and psychosocial factors affecting the lay definition of illness and the decision to use services. Such issues as ethnicity, household structure, values and attitudes, learned inclinations, informal influences, social distance, access to medical care, and situational stress have been identified as playing a role in the decision to consult a physician (Kasl and Cobb, 1966a, 1966b; Levine and Kozloff, 1978; Mechanic, 1978a:249–89; Robinson, 1971). In contrast, multivariate studies involving large samples and powerful statistical techniques find such factors, to the extent that they are included, relatively unimportant (Anderson et al., 1975; Kohn and White, 1976; Wolinsky, 1978; Aday and Eichhorn, 1972). One conclusion is that many medical sociologists have exaggerated the importance of social and organizational variables. A contrasting hypothesis is that the lack of such findings in the multivariate studies reflects the way issues are conceptualized, the nature of the measures used, the ways in which data are aggregated, and the manner in which analyses are performed. This paper examines these issues.

There is a major difference characterizing these two literatures. Illness-behavior studies are explicitly more theoretical, are more likely to involve small samples interviewed intensively, and include more qualitative assessment, emphasis on the subject's subjective understandings, and attention to social definitions and social processes over time. In contrast, the multivariate studies typically are based on a general conceptual scheme, involve large cross-sectional surveys, and use less detailed and more general measures to represent the concepts being studied. Different implications for the need to pay attention to sociocultural and psychosocial considerations in physician utilization emerge from these two approaches.

The issue extends well beyond the medical sociology literature. Economists and health services researchers, for example, have made a persuasive theoretical case and have generated much data showing relationships between the use of medical care and such factors as income, insurance coverage, and accessibility of providers (Fuchs, 1974; Klarman, 1965; Davis, 1975; Wennberg and Gittelsohn, 1973; Newhouse et al., 1974). Indeed, our entire understanding of the functioning of health services systems is premised on the common observation that increased insurance coverage and increased access to providers of care result in greater demand and use of services. Thus it is curious indeed that large-scale multivariate surveys fail to demonstrate the importance of variations in such factors. This paper explores why this might be the case. Although I suggest various possibilities, each having some bearing on the issue, taken singly or even in combination, they fail to provide a fully satisfactory explanation of the gaps that exist between these various literatures.

Multivariate Models of Physician Utilization

A conceptual approach developed by Andersen and his co-workers (Andersen et al., 1975; Aday and Andersen, 1975) to guide multivariate analyses, and used frequently by others, conceives of physician utilization as a consequence of predisposing, enabling, and illness (need) variables. *Predisposing* variables refer to those that exist prior to the onset of illness and include demographic factors (age and sex, for example), social structural variables (ethnicity, occupation, and education), and beliefs about medical care, physicians, and disease. *Enabling* factors "include family resources such as income and level of health insurance coverage or other source of third party payment, and the existence, nature and accessibility of a regular source of health care" (Andersen et al., 1975:6). Community characteristics such as number of health facilities and personnel, region, or rural-urban nature of the community may also be relevant as enabling variables.

Need is divided by Andersen et al. into perceived need and evaluated need. *Perceived* need is measured by (1) the number of reported bed days and other restricted activity days resulting from injury or illness, (2) number of symptoms reported from a checklist including such symptoms as "sudden feeling of weakness or faintness," "getting up some mornings tired and exhausted even with a usual amount of rest," "feeling tired for weeks at a time for no special reason," and "frequent headaches" (Aday and Andersen, 1975:84), and (3) self-perceived general state of health. *Evaluated* illness includes symptom scores weighted by the extent to which physicians indicated that persons should see a doctor for these symptoms and physicians' ratings of the medical severity of the diagnoses reported in the interview.

The studies by Andersen and his colleagues are examples of well-executed, large-scale physician utilization studies. They deal with nationally representative samples, make efforts to validate reports of utilization, introduce indicators of need for care as well as economic and social variables, and use sophisticated multivariate approaches in the analysis of results. The most extensively reported data come from a 1971 survey of 3,880 families comprising 11,822 persons. This sample was designed to ensure adequate representation of groups of special interest, such as rural residents, aged persons, and the inner-city poor.

When the descriptive model is applied to those data, however, it yields modest results whether predicting contact with a physician or volume of visits (Andersen et al., 1975). Using a large number of predictors, the model explains from 16% to 25% of the variance, but almost all of the variance explained results from perceived or evaluated illness variables. In the 1971 study, for example, 85% of the variance in physician contact explained is accounted for by three perceived illness variables: worry about health (7.6%), disability days (4.8%), and symptoms (1.4%). In the case of volume of visits, diagnostic severity and perceived illness account for almost all of the 23.4% of variance explained: severity of diagnosis (14%), disability days (4.6%), symptoms (1.9%), perceived health (1%), worry about health (0.7%), and pain frequency (0.7%). A sizeable effect of having a regular source of care is found on contact with a physician, but the remarkable fact is that the variance that can be explained by the other predisposing and enabling variables of Andersen et al, when perceived and evaluated illness variables are taken into account, is very small. Although they get somewhat varying results using Automatic Interaction Detection (AID) and Multiple Classification Analysis (MCA), the order of importance of predictors in the two analyses is similar.

In 1975-76 Andersen and Aday collected data from another national sample of 7,787 persons, with an 85% response rate. They report regression coefficients for number of physician visits involving a model with nine independent variables that account for 22% of the variance. Once again illness variables account for most of the variance explained; symptoms and perceived health yielded standardized beta coefficients of .32 and .19.

Having a usual source of care yielded a beta of .12, consistent with the findings of the 1971 survey (Andersen and Aday, 1978).

Another major empirical study of utilization, the International Collaborative Study (Kohn and White, 1976), examined predictors of physician contact within two weeks in 12 study areas in seven countries. Using Multiple Classification Analysis, the investigators considered a wide variety of predisposing factors, enabling factors, and illness variables. Using 21 predictors very much like those used by Andersen et al., and adopting a similar conceptual scheme, they were able to explain 4% to 10% of the variance in adult physician utilization in varying geographic areas. Predictability achieved by variables other than morbidity factors, either individually or in the aggregate, was trivial (Kohn and White, 1976:184–85). With the exception of perceived severity of illness, no other variable produced statistically significant results across areas.

Wolinsky (1978) attempted to predict physician utilization using the health interview survey for the years 1971 to 1973. He reports on regression models of physician visits in the prior 12 months and on length of interval since last physician visit using 29 predictors. These predictors explain from 9% to 12% of the variance in amount of utilization and from 14% to 16% in length of interval. Illness-morbidity measures account for most of the findings, although predisposing variables have some influence on the length-of-interval dependent variable. Wolinsky approaches these data in a less systematic way than is characteristic of the studies by Andersen and associates, and the "shotgun" analysis and the lack of any theoretical rationale make it difficult to interpret the findings. They are generally consistent, however, with other large-scale physician utilization studies.

Hershey et al. (1975) provide a more thoughtful approach in analyzing data from 315 families (including 1,065 individuals) in the San Joaquin Valley in California. They propose a behavioral model in which pathology results in the development of symptoms and wants culminating in demand for physician services. The available supply is seen as exerting an independent effect on utilization. The authors, however, distinguish various types of physician utilization, such as total outpatient visits, number of patient-initiated visits, and obtaining a checkup. They argue quite reasonably that one would anticipate different determinants of varying types of physician utilization, and compute separate regression equations for each type.

"Health status" measures and usual-source-of-care measures predicted all types of utilization, although "health status" was more important in predicting amount of utilization than whether a physician was seen at all or whether the patient had a checkup. Other variables, such as age, income, ethnicity, and education of head of family, were found to be important for some types of utilization. The major results, however, are basically consistent with those of Andersen's surveys, and in no case were attitudes such as self-reliance, fatalism, or ethnocentricity statistically significant predictors. Hershey et al. (1975:849) properly note that the size of any regression coefficient depends on the other variables that are in the model. Thus inclusion of insurance coverage or usual source of care will affect the coefficient for income, which is related to these variables. They, however, do not expand the implications of their discussion concerning the need for models of the way predisposing, enabling, and illness variables relate to one another.

The consistency of the results from these various surveys is remarkable, particularly because they are discrepant with the more qualitative literature in medical sociology and with much of the economic analysis of the effects of insurance coverage and resource availability on use of medical care. One possibility is that qualitative studies and more theoretically focused quantitative studies that limit the predictive variables used have exaggerated the impact of culture, ethnicity, accessibility, and attitudes, or have focused on spurious relationships resulting from the lack of proper controls. Although this hypothesis is probably true to some extent, it is not an adequate explanation.

If sociocultural factors and resource availability are not important, how can the vast differences in utilization across areas be explained? Physician utilization from one geographic area to another, and from one population group to another, may vary three- or fourfold, and international variations among populations in different nations may vary from an average of 2 visits to 10 or 12 visits. One possibility is that, because of increasing insurance coverage in the United States and programs such as Medicare and Medicaid, most of the population has reached the requisite threshold to obtain the number of physician visits necessary in relation to medical need. Although accessibility has substantially increased, it is unlikely to have brought everyone to a point where enabling variables would be expected to be irrelevant. Moreover, the enabling variables that Andersen and his associates used have respondents well distributed, suggesting that the lack of findings is not simply a result of a lack of heterogeneity in the population studied (Andersen et al., 1975:269–75). Thus the remainder of this paper examines from varying theoretical and methodological perspectives the reasons that these multivariate studies achieve such limited predictability.

The Interpretation of Morbidity Measures

A major difficulty in surveys of health is the inadequacy of questionnaire indicators of illness and health status. Although questions on perceived health status, symptoms, chronic disease, and restricted activity are commonly asked, these usually reflect a complex pattern of illness perception and behavior that goes beyond the narrower conceptual definition of morbidity that researchers would, ideally, like to measure. These proxy variables for measuring morbidity are often correlated with various sociodemographic, attitudinal, and behavioral variables, and when introduced into multiple regression equations reduce the influence of such predictors. Andersen et al., for example, note many such zero-order relationships (1975:14–15), although most have modest influence in relation to morbidity variables, but they are attenuated and lack statistical significance in the multivariate equations. One conception is that these are simply spurious associations; another is that they are determinative of a process of care masked by the multivariate procedures used. From a behavioral perspective, such variables as attention to pain, perception of health status, and release from usual activities should be seen not simply as indicators of illness but also as part of a dynamic process of interpretation and behavior. Examining such dynamic processes is likely to contribute meaningfully to social policy and to improving clinical practice.

One measure of "illness" typically used is respondents' perceptions of their health. Whereas physicians have been trained to identify discrete disease problems that they can manage in specific ways, patients tend to have a more global view. They react experientially to their overall sense of well-being and to the extent that their symptoms disrupt their ability to function or interfere with important life activities. In one analysis, Richard Tessler and I (1978) analyzed four diverse data sets to ascertain predictors of subjective health status. We studied samples of employed workers in two industries, a student population, a prison population, and a sample of persons aged 45 to 69 in a southern state. The purpose of these analyses was to examine the role of psychological distress in explaining subjective ill health when "actual health status" was controlled. Psychological distress was significantly associated with subjective ill health in all data sets. The ordering of the relationship, of course, can be interpreted either way. We also found that the more objective the "actual health status" control variable (as, for example, when a physician rating is used as compared with a list of chronic health problems), the larger the association.

In a more recent analysis I have examined predictors of subjective physical health status among 302 young adults who were first studied as children in 1961, and followed up in 1977 (Mechanic, 1978b, 1979). Among the most substantial predictors of perceived poor health status in 1977 were the respondent's report that the mother acknowledged more pain and discomfort and released herself from usual activities more readily when the child was 10 to 14 years old, the respondent's report that he or she gets sick easily, the respondent's report of more life problems causing worry, a low score on a scale of enjoying physical activity, low educational status, a low score on a scale of preventive medical care, more chronic health problems, and greater reported unhappiness. This reported perception thus seems to be in part learned in childhood, in part shaped by one's location in society, and in part conditioned by psychological stress. It is not simply an index of physical health.

The fact that such factors as social position and stress are important in the use of the physician is illustrated by Tessler et al. (1976) in a prospective study of physician utilization in a prepaid group practice. When "health status" was controlled, two factors that retained importance in predicting utilization were the respondents' prior state of psychological distress and sex. It is not surprising that large-scale multivariate studies may not find these factors influential in regression equations with many predictors. If the "illness measures" already encompass the sex and distress variance, they will diminish the relevant betas.

Consider the measures of number of symptoms (perceived illness) and evaluated symptoms used by Andersen et al. (1975). In both cases, the index is heavily weighted with symptom items commonly associated with psychological distress, e.g., headaches, tiredness, and weakness. Indeed these items occur so commonly in psychological disorder that they tend to be used as components of such measures as the Langner scale (Langner, 1962). They hardly can be considered valid measures of "illness" as the term is used in medical practice; many of the items resemble those used in general scales of well-being.

Another illness variable Andersen and his colleagues find to be important is worry about health, which accounts for 7.6% of the variance at the zero-order level in contact with physicians and 7.7% of the variance in volume of visits. In the child study referred to earlier, I have had some opportunity to examine this variable and find, as in the case of physical health ratings, that this measure is substantially related to various dimensions of psychological distress, such as unhappiness, reported distress, reported life problems causing worries, and low self-esteem. Similar problems pertain to limitation of usual activities when ill and bed disability. My longitudinal study of the development of health behavior patterns indicates that such limitations are learned in part and relate to health attitudes more generally. For example, young adults in 1977 who were more inclined to limit activities and seek release from usual obligations when ill had mothers in 1961 who also limited activities when ill and who were low on a scale of personal control over illness. Such release from usual obligations was also related to more health concern and a lower assessment of one's health, less happiness, and a lower score on a risk-taking attitude scale.

The one measure used by Andersen and his colleagues (Andersen et al., 1975) that approaches more clearly the concept of the nature and severity of disease is physician judgments of patient diagnoses. This measure is not used in the analysis of physician contact because there can be no evaluation of diagnoses for persons who did not visit a physician. In explaining volume of visits, however, it accounts for 14% of the variance, three-fifths of all variance explained. The analysis of volume of visits excludes those not using a physician at all.

Kravits and Schneider (1975:173–74) provide a detailed discussion of the construction of this complex diagnosis measure. Patient diagnoses are first coded into a modified classification-of-disease scheme combined with a rating of severity. These are then assigned to four categories by physicians: (1) preventive care or care from a physician would make no difference, (2) symptomatic relief could be obtained from a physician, (3) the person should see a doctor, and (4) the person must see a doctor. Because individuals may have more than one diagnosis, each individual is then assigned to one of three categories that constitute the final measure: (A) elective care only (codes 1 or 2), (B) both elective and mandatory care (codes 1 or 2 *and* 3 or 4), and (C) mandatory care only (codes 3 or 4).

An analysis of the diagnosis measure indicates that its construction involves several levels of decision-making, each of which may introduce complexities in interpretation. Because record verification of reported diagnoses could be obtained for only 58% of physician contacts, coding must depend on the way respondents report their illness, which may involve differential illness perceptions and behavior. Physician coding decisions also are highly judgmental and dependent on the quality of data provided. One potential problem with this measure is that persons who visit the physician only infrequently may be disproportionately assigned to code "A." Although some making only one visit may receive both elective and mandatory care during that visit, it is likely that those assigned to code "B" will pay more than one visit, given the procedures used for coding. Thus the coding procedure may produce a redundancy between the independent and dependent variables, and an unknown amount of the predictability of the diagnosis variable may be a product of this redundancy. Reanalysis of the data would be necessary to determine the extent of bias introduced by this coding method.

What has been said about the study by Andersen and his colleagues is even more true of the International Utilization Study and other large-scale studies. Andersen et al. are exemplary in that they carefully attempted to develop independent need measures, a difficult procedure at best. The practical difficulty of doing this results in a reliance on perceived levels of health in most other studies, including the International Study. The key point is not that the data are in question, but that it is difficult to interpret them clearly. The discussion of concept measurement and aggregation of data that follows raises other types of issues.

Problems of Concept Measurement and Data Aggregation

One of the puzzling aspects of the findings from large-scale physician utilization studies is the lack of support for the importance of enabling family and community variables, such as family income, insurance, residence, region, and M.D.-to-population ratio. Regular source of care, the only significant variable of this kind, explained 2.4% of the variation in contact with a physician in the AID analysis carried out by Andersen and his colleagues (1975:16–17). Because regular source of care is associated to some extent with other enabling variables, this may partly account for the lack of positive findings. Andersen and Aday's (1978) analysis of their 1975–76 data, however, suggests that this explanation is not a satisfactory one. Age, race, education, family income, doctor visit insurance, and M.D.-to-population ratio accounted for only 4% of the variation in regular source of care, and the zero-order correlations are small.

The small effect of a measure such as doctor visit insurance on physician utilization is highly inconsistent with observations and estimates of the impact of physician ambulatory care coverage on the demand for medical care (Newhouse et al., 1974). One problem in defining these predictors is the lack of precise specification of the independent variable. The measure of insurance coverage, for example, simply distinguishes between no insurance, basic coverage, and major medical and fails to note degree of coverage or the amount of coinsurance and deductibles. The measure of the M.D. office coverage variable involves simply a yes-no response and fails to elicit the nature and extent of coverage. Existing theory would argue, in contrast, that what must be understood is the magnitude of economic barriers as measured by the requirement for out-of-pocket expenditures.

In the case of such variables as residence, region, and M.D.-to-population ratio, the predictors are crude categorizations. M.D. ratio, for example, is computed on the basis of the population of the SMSA or rural county of family residence (Andersen et al., 1975:278). One would anticipate, however, that such factors as physician ratio, which is an indirect measure of access, would have to be computed on the basis of the population of small geographic areas to capture adequately the behavioral consequences of varying resource availability. Many urban inner-city areas or rural populations with low physician access may be in SMSAs or counties with a high M.D.-to-population ratio. Using aggregated population indices for large areas is unlikely to capture the natural opportunities and constraints for small subgroups of the population. Yet, having said all this, it is still curious that the crude categorizations depict so little variation. Davis (1975), in a study of benefit utilization under Medicare, found fairly substantial associations between physician utilization and race, region, income, and available physicians. Her data referred only to persons over 65 years of age, and some of her largest findings involved interaction terms such as blacks in the South. Given the heterogeneous population covered by the large national samples, however, it is intriguing that they note so few effects of enabling variables.

Cross-Sectional Versus Processual Studies

A major contrast between many micro-level studies of medical care utilization and the cross-sectional multivariate studies is the underlying conception of the way physician utilization is triggered. A common theoretical view in the general medical-sociological literature is that utilization results from a subtle definitional and interactional process through which persons become aware of a need, appraise the nature of that need in relation to competing needs and definitions, examine alternative solutions, and in some fashion weigh the costs and benefits of such solutions. The final decision may be dependent on the nature of the appraisal, available competing definitions, interpersonal needs and influences, and situational contingencies.

The underlying argument is that the determinants of help-seeking are part of a dynamic process involving response and feedback from the environment and cannot be simply abstracted through general descriptors of the persons involved or their environments. In theory, people with identical symptoms might behave differently depending on what is going on in their lives and on situational factors, and this cannot be captured through cross-sectional study. Proponents of this view would argue that the modest amount of variance explained in large-scale multivariate studies, even when a large number of predictor variables are used, reflects the nature of the data and the limitations of the method.

The qualitative studies of illness response and behavior focus on the processes of identification and definition and the way they are influenced by culture, stress, and interpersonal factors. Zola (1966), for example, has noted marked differences in perceptions and responses among Irish and Italian patients and maintains that it is "this selective process and not an etiological one which accounts for the many unexplained or over-explained epidemiological differences observed between and within societies" (Zola, 1966:619). Robinson (1971), in an intensive study of the illness behavior of 24 families, notes that "just as some people, because of the particular demands of their social positions, were more likely than others to consider a particular sign to be a symptom of illness so, in response to the demands of adequately performing certain social roles, the symptomatic person and various significant others may differ in their readiness to allow the symptomatic person legitimate access to the status sick" (p. 110). Roghmann and Haggerty (1975), in studying the relationship between stress, illness, and medical utilization, note the importance of proximity in time between such links and suggest "that the clustering of events over time is a stochastic process that may approach the model of a regular Markov chain" (p. 147).

The analytic issues raised by different types of strategies for studying physician utilization are not unique to this area. Svarstad (1976), for example, in studying patient conformity with medical advice, notes inconsistencies in the research literature on such varied factors as sex, age, income, education, occupation, race, family structure, attitudes, intelligence, and personality factors. She observes that in contrast to the assumptions underlying this literature, patients do not behave consistently across situations; their behavior varies from one time to another and may vary by the nature of instruction and types of advice. She argues that "focusing on the *process* by which nonconformity is prevented and reduced may be more productive than concentrating on individual characteristics" (p. 221). She then provides a brilliant analysis of the instruction process in relation to patient adherence based on observing doctor-patient interactions and interviewing patients a week later.

Other Approaches to Physician Utilization

In addition to multivariate approaches already described, a variety of other models have been suggested that focus to a larger extent on sociocultural and social-psychological issues. Antonovsky (1972), for example, suggests a model in which he includes host characteristics, characteristics of the medical institutions, and characteristics of the larger sociocultural environment. Host characteristics include latent need, intolerance of ambiguity of symptoms, and an orientation toward the use of professionals; medical systems variables include availability of facilities, the ability of medical institutions to be responsive to various latent functions, and the degree of receptivity of physicians; and the sociocultural environment variables include organizational facilitation in using medical services, absence of stigma for such use, cultural pressures to have problems diagnosed, and the degree of availability of functional alternatives.

Antonovsky's model takes account of the fact that medical care constitutes a small social system that may be used to deal with diffuse social and psychological needs when the system is available, when its use is socially encouraged, and when it is receptive to peoples' needs and orientations. One study examining some aspects of this model in Israel, which has a population with high social need and a high physician-patient ratio, found that higher levels of need for catharsis, legitimation of failure, and the resolution of the magic-science conflict were associated with higher levels of utilization (Shuval, 1970). Another study in Israel by Mann and colleagues (1970) found that latent social need was influential in the long-term pattern of use of health services. Persons who had been in concentration camps had much higher levels of physician utilization over a period of years that could not be accounted for solely on the basis of illness patterns.

The research on social need points to the fact that the provision of medical care is not simply a socioeconomic process, but is also an important aspect of social adaptation. We have ample evidence that there is large overlap between the occurrence of illness in populations that does not result in utilization of the physician and the most common presenting complaints seen by the physician of first contact. The main task for the behavioral scientist is to understand why persons with similar complaints behave so differently and why the same person with comparable symptoms at various times choose to seek medical care on one occasion but not on another (Mechanic, 1978a). Such processes depend on a wide range of factors, as the medical sociology literature suggests, including the organization of physician services and the receptivity of health personnel to varying types of problems and to sociocultural alternatives to medical care. Many of the large-scale utilization studies are not designed with the intention of elucidating these processes. However, a careful dissection is required of the ways in which people perceive their bodies, make sense of their symptoms, and come to depend on the medical care system. Safer et al. (1979), for example, have provided data in support of the argument that the determinants of illness appraisal, decisions to seek care, and physician utilization are different and should be studied as separate stages.

A variety of models of illness behavior have been suggested (Zola, 1964; Mechanic, 1978a:249–89; Rosenstock, 1969). These models take into account the relationships between perceptions of illness and social functioning needs as well as such issues as attribution of cause and risks and benefits of treatment. Although these models direct attention to more subtle processes of perception and definition, they are difficult to test in large-scale surveys of a cross-sectional nature. Thus these models tend to be tested in only one aspect or another, making it difficult to establish the degree of redundancy between different types of predictors described in the literature.

Conclusions

As this discussion suggests, there is a wide gap between two literatures dealing with physician utilization. Even though these contrasting types of studies are designed to address different substantive and policy questions, the contradictions in findings are disconcerting. Although it is difficult to understand all of the discrepant results, many of them are accounted for by the types of populations studied, the definitions of variables, the analytic strategies used, and the manner in which data are aggregated. Both types of studies offer distinctive advantages, and ideally the advantages of both can be combined in future research strategies.

The benefits of the large-scale surveys include the size and representativeness of the samples studied, the range of variables included, and the ability to introduce statistical controls to identify spurious findings. In contrast, the traditional studies provide a richer view of perceptions and reactions and a better conception of social process, and are more able to capture the link between events, perceptions, and utilization within a single behavioral sequence. It would be useful, although reasonably difficult, to examine various psychosocial hypotheses that emerge from the qualitative studies with a broad multivariate design. Ideally, such a study would be prospective, would gather information from the same respondents at various intervals, and would at least obtain detailed qualitative information from a subsample to help enrich our understanding of the behavioral processes involved. As a start, it would be useful in bringing these two literatures together to recognize that what are characterized as "illness" variables in the multivariate studies are more appropriately seen as illness-behavior measures incorporating various learned inclinations, value orientations, and life events as well as physical illness.

The traditional medical sociology literature on physician utilization would be enriched by examining psychosocial processes within an economic context that takes into account enabling variables such as access to care, the availability of providers, and scope of insurance coverage. Examining the role of cultural and social-psychological processes within the constraining influences of economic and organizational factors will result in better theory and, it is to be hoped, more adequate prediction.

References

Aday, LuAnn, and Ronald Andersen
1975   Development of Indices of Access to Medical Care. Ann Arbor: Health Administration Press.

Aday, Lu Ann, and Robert Eichhorn
1972   The Utilization of Health Services: Indices and Correlates. A Research Bibliography, 1972. National Center for Health Services Research and Development, DHEW Pub. No. (HSM) 73-3003.

Andersen, R., and L. A. Aday
1978   "Access to medical care in the U.S.: Realized and potential." Medical Care 16:533–46.

Andersen, Ronald, Joanna Kravits, and Odin W. Anderson (eds.)
1975   Equity in Health Services: Empirical Analyses in Social Policy. Cambridge: Ballinger.

Antonovsky, A.
1972   "A model to explain visits to the doctor: With specific reference to the case of Israel." Journal of Health and Social Behavior 13:466–54.

Davis, K.
1975   "Equal treatment and unequal benefits: The Medicare program." The Milbank Memorial Fund Quarterly (Health and Society) 53:449–88.

Fuchs, Victor R.
1974   Who Shall Live? Health, Economics, and Social Choice. New York: Basic Books.

Hershey, J. C., H. S. Luft, and J. M. Gianaris
1975   "Making sense out of utilization data." Medical Care 13:838–54.

Kasl, S. V. and S. Cobb
1966a   "Health behavior, illness behavior, and sick role behavior: I. Health and illness behavior." Archives of Environmental Health 12:246–66.
1966b   "Health behavior, illness behavior, and sick-role behavior: II. Sick-role behavior." Archives of Environmental Health 12:531–41.

Klarman, Herbert E.
1965   The Economics of Health. New York: Columbia University Press.

Kohn, Robert, and Kerr L. White (eds.)
1976   Health Care—An International Study: Report of the World Health Organization/International Collaborative Study of Medical Care Utilization. London: Oxford University Press.

Kravits, J., and J. Schneider
1975   "Health care need and actual use by age, race and income." Pp. 169–87 in Ronald Andersen, Joanna Kravits, and Odin W. Anderson (eds.), Equity in Health Services: Empirical Analyses in Social Policy. Cambridge: Ballinger.

Langner, T. S.
1962   "A twenty-two item screening score of psychiatric symptoms indicating impairment." Journal of Health and Human Behavior 3:269–76.

Levine, S., and M. A. Kozloff
   1978   "The sick role: Assessment and overview." Annual Review of Sociology (Palo Alto, Cal.) 4:317–43.

Mann, K. J., Jack H. Medalie, Elinor Lieber, J. J. Groen, and Louis Guttman
   1970   Visits to Doctors. Jerusalem: Jerusalem Academic Press.

Mechanic, David
   1978a   Medical Sociology, 2nd ed. New York: Free Press.
   1978b   "Correlates of health and illness behavior: Results from a 16-year follow-up." Research and Analytic Report Series No. 8–78. Center for Medical Sociology and Health Services Research, University of Wisconsin, Madison.
   1979   "Correlates of psychological distress among young adults: A theoretical hypothesis and results from a 16-year follow-up study." Research and Analytic Report Series No. 1–79, Center for Medical Sociology and Health Services Research, University of Wisconsin, Madison.

Newhouse, J. P., C. E. Phelps, and W. B. Schwartz
   1974   "Policy options and the impact of national health insurance." New England Journal of Medicine 290:1345–59.

Robinson, David
   1971   The Process of Becoming Ill. London: Routledge and Kegan Paul.

Roghmann, K. J., and R. J. Haggerty
   1975   "The stress model for illness behavior." Pp. 142–56 in Robert J. Haggerty, Klaus J. Roghmann, and Ivan B. Pless (eds.), Child Health and the Community. New York: Wiley-Interscience.

Rosenstock, I. M.
   1969   "Prevention of illness and maintenance of health." Pp. 168–90 in John Kosa, Aaron Antonovsky, and Irving Kenneth Zola (eds.), Poverty and Health: A Sociological Analysis. Cambridge: Harvard University Press.

Safer, M. A., Q.J . Tharps, T. C. Jackson, and H. Leventhal
   1979   "Determinants of three stages of delay in seeking care at a medical-clinic." Medical Care 17:11–29.

Shuval, Judith T., in collaboration with Aaron Antonovsky and A. Michael Davies
   1970   Social Functions of Medical Practice. San Francisco: Jossey-Bass.

Svarstad, B. L.
   1976   "Physician-patient communication and patient conformity with medical advice." Pp. 220–38 in David Mechanic, The Growth of Bureaucratic Medicine: An Inquiry into the Dynamics of Patient Behavior and the Organization of Medical Care. New York: Wiley-Interscience.

Tessler, R., and D. Mechanic
   1979   "Psychological distress and perceived health status." Journal of Health and Social Behavior 19:254–62.

Tessler, R., D. Mechanic, and M. Dimond
   1976   "The effect of psychological distress on physician utilization: A prospective study."Journal of Health and Social Behavior 17:353–64.

Wennberg, J., and A. Gittelsohn
   1973   "Small area variations in health care delivery." Science 182:1102–8.

Wolinsky, F. D.
    1978   "Assessing the effects of predisposing, enabling, and illness-morbidity characteristics on health service utilization." Journal of Health and Social Behavior 19:384–96.

Zola, I. K.
    1964   "Illness behavior of the working class: Implications and recommendations." Pp. 350–61 in Arthur B. Shostak and William Gomberg (eds.), Blue-Collar World: Studies of the American Worker. Englewood Cliffs, N.J.: Prentice-Hall.
    1966   "Culture and symptoms—An analysis of patients' presenting complaints." American Sociological Review 31:615–30.

10

Development of Psychological Distress among Young Adults

There is a vast literature in psychiatric epidemiology on the occurrence of symptoms of psychological and psychophysiological distress in community and patient populations of various kinds.[1,2] A number of interview or questionnaire scales have been developed in recent decades, influenced by the Neuropsychiatric Screening Questionnaire.[3] Such instruments as the Langner 22-item scale,[4] the Gurin Mental Status Index,[5] and the Health Opinion Survey[6] have been used to screen community populations for psychological disorder, and similarly the Cornell Medical Index[7] has been used in screening medical outpatient populations. Despite decades of serious effort, there is great difficulty in knowing how to interpret the scores obtained from these instruments and their conceptual relationships to illness concepts and clinical judgments.

Although clinical populations score higher on these scales than community samples, there are a variety of anomalies that alert concern about what these scales really measure. Psychiatric outpatients, for example, score higher on psychiatric screening items than more seriously disabled inpatients,[8] and average scores are high among normal competent youth, such as university students.[9] Comparisons of scores obtained on two occasions among community samples and patients find much greater stability among patients,[8] suggesting that in one context the scales may measure enduring states while in another may measure relatively transient ones. Also, comparisons of psychiatric clinical judgments and research diagnostic criteria with symptom profiles derived from these questionnaires show considerable disagreement in the identification of cases.[10,11]

Dohrenwend developed five scales to measure distinct dimensions of psychopathology, including the types of items in typical screening interviews, and found them to be reliable in varying subgroups, correlated with quality of functioning, and capable of discriminating psychiatric patients from normal populations (unpublished data). However, he found that these scales measure a single common dimension, only poorly related to clinical concepts of psychiatric disorder. In an epidemiological study in Marshfield, Wis, with 1,512 respondents, which my colleagues and I are conducting, considerable effort has been made to develop varying scales of psychopathology consistent with clinical concepts and using many of Dohrenwend's items. These scales, however, tend to be highly correlated and most are substantially correlated with the Langner 22-item scale. For example, the Langner score was correlated with the following scales: manic (.47), thinking disturbance (.69), delusions (.46), explosiveness (.43), anxiety (.87), fears (.55), guilt (.68), sadness (.73), hopelessness (.74), suicide (.47), enervation (.72), boredom (.45), withdrawal (.33), sleep problems (.66), psychophysiological symptoms (.79), perception of physical condition (.55), possibly psychogenic (.69), low self-esteem (.48), suspicion (.62), obsessive neurotic (.38), and Eysenck's neuroticism scale (.63). Langner scores were also correlated (− .47) with perceived disability.

The issue remains: what do these symptom instruments measure? Dohrenwend (in an unpublished manuscript) addresses this question in some detail, reviewing various explanations: that these scales measure neurosis; that they reflect a particular mode of expression in which the individual reports dissatisfaction mainly within him or herself; that the scales measure something akin to fever in physical illness; or that they measure a "pseudo or quasi neurosis" reflecting psychological discomfort and maladjustment. Dohrenwend finds all these concepts wanting, adopting Frank's[12] concept of demoralization—a situation in which a person cannot meet expectations, but also cannot escape. Dohrenwend notes the following:

> Among the sources of the predicament Frank mentions environmental stresses, giving the example of wartime experiences; constitutional defects; learned incapacity; existential despair; all physical illnesses, especially chronic physical illnesses; and "crippling [psychiatric] symptoms." Clearly, Frank's theoretical formulation of the construct "demoralization" fits the facts discovered and questions raised in the present study leading to our composite scale of psychological-and-somatic distress and the results obtained by others with screening scales that are similar to it.

The issue of what these scales measure is important because patients with similar types of generalized complaints come frequently to psychiatrists, primary care physicians, emergency rooms, hospital outpatient departments, counselors, and a variety of other helping sources and social agencies. Moreover, the evidence of high rates of such symptoms in community populations is often used as justification for extending services.[13] Although the concept of demoralization covers the range of symptoms measured by such scales, it is more descriptive than theoretical, and while Frank suggests a variety of causes of demoralization, his discussion of its development, other than in such cases as thought reform and religious conversion, is vague.

Frank's discussion of demoralization is a valuable place to begin, but it is only one aspect of a complex pattern of illness behavior[14] that combines psychological and physical symptomatology with cultural definitions and meanings, personal response inclinations, and situational pressures. After presenting a theoretical hypothesis of the way such patterns may develop, I examine various data from a 16-year prospective study that allow some consideration of the role of developmental factors in the emergence of such distress syndromes. Although this study was not designed specifically to examine the issues raised here, it provides some unique data.

A Theoretical Hypothesis

The concept of psychological distress as used in this report is a general expression of suffering and probably reflects a variety of influences, including psychiatric disorder and situational stress. The hypothesis to be examined is that such responses can best be viewed as a latent expressive mode first shaped in childhood but elaborated on throughout a person's developmental history. Many factors may contribute to personal suffering, but the perception and expression of that pain are molded by meanings people learn to assign to inner feeling states and the extent to which they focus on them and monitor them. The measured distress response, it is argued, is a combination of objective and subjective, symptoms and definitions, and illness and illness behavior. The meanings attributed to pain and how it is expressed are shaped by family life and the sociocultural context.

In an earlier analysis,[15] I suggested that the definition of illness was shaped by three aspects: bodily sensations, symptoms, or feelings different from usual; social stress; and cognitive definitions that suggested organizing hypotheses about what the person is feeling. Changes in body sensations increase self-awareness, and stress contributes to body arousal and psychological disorientation that further motivate attention to inner feelings. Symptoms or feeling states may be redefined under stress or when new interpretive schemas are suggested. Typically, socialization has prepared us with conventional schemas by which we explain varying symptoms and feelings as when we attribute fatigue to a hard day's work or feelings of depression to a significant disappointment. When persons feel aroused, however, and when symptoms are not easily explained within conventional and commonly available understandings, external cues become important in establishing meaning. Such cues may be accidental, or they may be a consequence of unique prior experience or cultural learning.

Illness reactions are shaped over time depending on the occurrence of illness, learning and social experience, and environmental contingencies. Perhaps it is the complexity of the shaping of such reactions, and the multiple factors involved, that has made it so difficult to identify empirically developmental precursors of adult psychopathology, but the fact is that we have little to show for decades of effort on developmental study of adult neurosis.[16-18] Here I hypothesize that the distress syndrome that we often call "neurosis" and that Dohrenwend calls demoralization, is in part a learned pattern of illness behavior involving an intense focus on internal feeling states, careful monitoring of body sensations, and a high level of self-awareness. I suggest that this pattern is reinforced by childhood illness, parental behavior, and adverse life events.

The Research Context

Some suggestive data come from a 16-year follow-up study of children's health responses. In 1961, a sample of mother-child pairs was selected from the population of Madison, Wis, and independent data were obtained from mothers, children, teachers, and official school records. In addition, 198 mothers completed daily illness diaries for 15 days following their interview. The initial sample of children was selected to ensure a range of social class background and two age levels. Students in the study were selected from seven Madison schools in various areas of the city. The final sample included all fourth-grade children in five schools and one half of the eighth-grade students chosen randomly from the three middle schools in the city. The socioeconomic distributions of the fourth- and eighth-grade populations were substantially the same. The sample of 350 mother-child pairs constitutes 93% of the eligible sample population. Mothers were interviewed at home, while information from the children was obtained in school. Findings of the 1961 phase of the study are reported elsewhere.[19-21]

In 1977 a follow-up study of the 350 children in the 1961 sample was initiated. With the use of a variety of tracing techniques, 333 of these respondents were located (95%). Of the remaining 17, six had died and 11 could not be found. Of those located, 302 (91%) completed detailed questionnaires concerning their health and illness attitudes and values and their experience and behavior in relation to health concerns. Longitudinal studies are constrained by the types of information initially collected. Over time, theoretical and methodological issues change, and although the 1961 study was unique in that it focused on health concerns, in retrospect there were many important questions that were omitted. The questionnaire used in the 1977 study was a compromise between retaining comparability with questions asked in 1961 and the introduction of improved questionnaire items and new concerns. In the presentation of results, not only are findings relevant to the suggested theoretical approach reported, but also other relationships that may be of interest to readers who may wish to suggest alternative theoretical conceptions.

The Dependent Variable:
Psychological Distress

The dependent variable is based on a summative index of adult reports of the frequency of seven symptoms during the prior three months: loneliness, nervousness, feeling depressed or blue, didn't have the energy needed, feeling so restless couldn't sit long in a chair, feeling you couldn't take care of things because you couldn't get going, and felt you were going to have a nervous breakdown. These items are commonly used in scales of psychological disorder, distress, and depression, and when combined into a scale achieve a reasonable level of reliability (α = .80). The scale was not significantly correlated with sex ($-.05$). It had an average correlation of .56 with five other variables used in the study to tap lack of psychological well-being: self-description of unhappiness (.46), description of low spirits ($-.44$), degree of worry about eight specified life problems (.56), high neuroticism on Eysenck's scale (.77), and low self-esteem ($-.59$). It is also correlated .41 with the respondents' reports in 1977 that they had emotional problems, nervous trouble, or chronic nerves. In short, although somewhat different than the screening instruments used in community surveys, it is very comparable to them in item content and patterns of relationships.

One deterrent to prediction of distress in young adulthood on the basis of developmental factors is instability in the dependent measure. Studies of the Langner 22-item scale or subsets of items from this scale suggest that the three-to four-year correlation of scores on such scales is approximately .5 to .6.[22] The size of the correlation will, of course, be affected by both reliability problems and lack of stability. While we do not know the degree of stability that might exist over a 16-year period (the time span of the present study), it is unlikely to be as high as .50. As a result, it is more difficult to identify 1961 predictors of psychological distress in early adulthood.

In presenting some findings I depend on regression analysis. The data most suitable for causal analysis are those collected in 1961, 16 years prior to the measurement of adult psychological distress. Some retrospective reports of respondents concerning parents' health and illness behavior, their parents' behavior toward them, and their feelings about their parents are also briefly considered. Because such perceptions are likely to have been distorted by time and by life events, they receive only passing comment here.

Correlates of Distress in Young Adulthood

Relationships Between Physical and Psychological Symptoms

Most survey instruments measuring psychological symptoms are correlated with indices of bodily complaints. Studies of perceived physical health status among population groups also show that such subjective appraisals are correlated with psychological distress.[23,24] In the 1977 questionnaire, the respondent's distress score was correlated .29 with a subjective appraisal of poorer health; .42 with frequency of 15 physical symptoms in the three months prior to interview; .20 with a scale based on the presence in the previous year of 24 chronic health problems (two of which referred to emotional problems and chronic disease which may confound the relationship); and .19 with the frequency of worrying about one's health. Distress was also correlated .15 with the reported number of days in bed in the three months prior to interview because of illness. All of the above correlations are statistically significant at the .05 level. In short, findings within the sample are consistent with the literature more generally.

Unfortunately, we did not obtain data in 1961 on psychological distress in children, but in any case such distress is often masked through physical complaints and disruptive or withdrawing behavior and is difficult to measure reliably. We did, however, obtain measures of physical symptoms in childhood, and we assume on the basis of the literature that they may be linked to distress.

Early Experience

Our working hypothesis suggested that the tendency for children to learn to focus on bodily complaints would depend on illness experience as children. Presumably, children who experienced illness more commonly would learn to focus more on their internal states, which would in part shape adult monitoring behavior and result in greater sensitivity to internal feelings. Adult distress scores were significantly associated with the following 1961 indicators: the mother's report of the frequency her child had 11 acute physical symptoms such as headaches, sore throats, and vomiting (.19); her report of the frequency her child had headaches and indigestion (.16); the child's report in 1961 of not feeling like doing much when having pain ($-$.12); the teacher's rating of the child as less stoical than most children in respect to pain ($-$.15); and more days absent from school (abstracted from school district records) in 1959 (.18), 1961 (.14), 1962 (.12), and the total period of 1959 through 1962 (.19). In the 1961 study, 189 mothers of children also included in the follow-up study maintained illness diaries for 15 days in which they recorded symptoms and illnesses of various family members. The number of symptoms reported for the study child in 1961 was significantly correlated with adult distress (.17). The above findings suggest a link between early acute physical illness and later distress, but also suggest that some of the patterns of illness response in children may have already been in part established by the time we gathered the initial data. Elsewhere, I have reported sex differentiation in illness responses among these children in the fourth grade.[19]

In the initial interviews with mothers we obtained various information concerning their own symptoms, responses to illness, and responses to their children's illnesses. We would not anticipate these measures to have direct effects on adulthood distress. A few findings are worth noting, however, although only indirectly relevant to the theoretical formulation. Adulthood distress was significantly associated with the mother's report that her spouse shared little responsibility in 18 areas of family life ($-$.16) and her score on a scale indicating a lower tendency to go to the doctor in specified hypothetical situations ($-$.16).

The finding that adulthood distress was associated with mothers' low tendency to go to the doctor in 1961 was not anticipated, but is consistent with findings of other investigators. Kerckhoff and Back[25] used a similar hypothetical index in a study of the diffusion among female employees of a southern mill of a hysterical illness alleged to be caused by an unknown insect. They found that those with the alleged illness were under high strain but reported a low tendency to go to the doctor. They suggest that the hysterical condition was most likely to strike those women under strain who could not admit they had a problem and who did not know how to cope with it.

The 1961 predictors are intercorrelated to varying degrees, but four yield significant β coefficients when they are included together in a regression equation. Reestimation of the equation with these four variables (mother's report that her spouse shares less responsibility; mother's report of a lower tendency to go to the doctor; the frequency of the child's physical symptoms in 1961; and total days absent from school) yield a multiple correlation of .31 with a corrected coefficient of determination of 9% (see model 1 in Table 10.1).

The relationship between adult distress and childhood physical symptoms might reflect, of course, the psychological state of the child, which we did not measure. Children, however, complain frequently of stomachaches and headaches, and it has been suggested that such complaints are often an expression of psychosocial stress[26] more so than other common childhood acute complaints such as coughs or sore throats. Thus we constructed a separate index of the frequency of children's headaches and indigestion, as reported by the mothers in 1961, on the assumption that such symptoms might be more highly correlated with adult distress than the more diverse childhood symptomatology index. The correlation with distress, however, using the more restricted index was .16, as compared with .19 for the broader acute symptom index, providing little support for the assumption.

An alternative explanation to the one suggested for the link between childhood acute physical symptoms and illness behavior (school absence) to adult psychological distress is simply that certain children are constitutionally weaker and continue to be so, and thus sickly children become sickly adults. Several observations would go against this interpretation. The types of childhood symptoms measured (headaches, coughs, chills, sore throats, muscular aches and pains, indigestion, diarrhea, constipa-

TABLE 10.1
Regression Models Describing Predictors of Adulthood Distress

	β Coefficients		
	Model 1	Model 2	Model 3
1961 variables			
Frequency of child's physical symptoms	.12*	.13*	.10
Total days absent from school, 1959–1962	.14*	.15*	.12*
Mother's report that spouses share household responsibilities	−.16*	−.19*	−.14*
Mother's report of tendency to use physician services	−.13*	−.13*	−.09*
Response bias measures			
Social desirability response score	...	−.20*	−.17*
Score on complaining index	...	.19*	.14*
Measure of introspectiveness, introspective score	...	...	.39*
Multiple correlation	.31	.42	.57
Corrected coefficient of determination, %	9	16	30

*P significant at the .05 level.

tion, vomiting, skin rashes, and swelling) are not particularly indicative of serious childhood or chronic illness. Moreover, Lewis and his colleagues[26] have repeatedly examined young children who reported many acute illness complaints to a self-initiated nurse practitioner clinic established as part of a school experimental program. Monitoring utilization over a six-year period, they found that the vast majority of high complainers were high users throughout the six years. These children, however, were not sickly children; indeed, children with chronic illnesses such as diabetes tended to use the health service only to a moderate degree according to C. E. Lewis (written communication, Jan 12, 1979). Lewis and colleagues, on the basis of the materials they collected, believe that high complainers learn to use symptoms as modes of coping with psychosocial problems and that such illness behavior tends to be reinforced by parents, teachers, and health personnel. Similar observations have been noted in the case of children brought to child guidance clinics; although the symptoms presented were often common among untreated children of comparable age, it was the poor coping capacities of the mother that differentiated those brought for care.[27]

The observed link between childhood illness and adulthood distress could still be a result of a segment of sickly persons in the sample who became sick in childhood and remain sickly in young adulthood. In the follow-up respondents were asked if they had any serious illnesses when growing up, and about one fifth of the respondents reported such illnesses. Few were serious chronic illnesses, and pneumonia was the most common illness report. As for hospitalizations, the vast majority were for tonsillectomies; and appendicitis, pneumonia, and trauma as a result of accidents were also relatively common reasons for hospitalization. Neither reporting a serious illness ($r = .04$) nor being hospitalized as a child ($r = -.06$) was significantly associated with adulthood distress. This suggests that frequency of symptoms may be more important than serious sickness in attuning the child to inner feelings. The size of the correlation between acute physical symptoms and adulthood distress was comparable among those reporting a serious illness ($r = .15$) and those who did not ($r = .19$). However, the correlation between frequency of acute physical illness and adulthood distress was higher among children who were hospitalized ($r = .27$) as compared with those who were not ($r = .15$). Because most of these children had tonsillectomies, it is reasonable to assume that they more frequently had tonsillitis and middle ear infections as well. It is conceivable that the hospital experience highlights the importance of symptoms, thus reinforcing internal monitoring more among those who have more symptoms.

To pursue the issue further, the correlates of the frequency of childhood acute physical symptoms were examined. They suggest the childhood acute illness scale represents a developing pattern of illness behavior more than serious illness. Children with more acute physical symptoms in 1961 were more likely to report at the time that they get sick easily (.25) and to be absent from school ($r = .44$ with school attendance 1959 through 1962). Teachers were also likely to characterize such children as having a poor ability to resist illness ($-.26$), as complainers when they had slight symptoms (.18), as less stoical than average ($-.14$), and as hypochondriacal (.16). Having many acute physical symptoms was only modestly associated with retrospective reports of having had a serious illness as a child (.12) or being hospitalized as a child (.19). Children having more acute symptoms were more likely to be in fourth as compared with eighth grade ($-.14$) and to have younger mothers ($-.14$).

When mothers were interviewed in 1961, they were asked about frequency of personal problems during the previous six months in relation to worrying, difficulties with spouse, difficulties with children, difficulties with relatives, inability to sleep, indigestion, nervousness, difficulties with duties, headaches, allergies, and feelings of depression. A problem score based on this heterogeneous group of items was correlated .27 with the children's acute physical symptoms reported by the mother. Mothers who reported more acute physical complaints for their children were also more likely to report that they did not enjoy their usual obligations (.12) and greater readiness to allow the child to go to school with various symptoms (.14). In contrast these mothers reported a greater inclination to give medication to the children when they had various symptoms (.16). Mothers who report more acute physical illness in their children report more disagreement with their spouses on family roles and relationships (.16), as well as more nervousness and depression (.22).

The picture that emerges from this pattern of correlations is that mothers who report more acute physical symptoms in their children are more troubled persons who are experiencing more family difficulties and are having more physical symptoms, problems, and dissatisfactions. The family climate might be characterized as involving considerable tension, with the mother attentive to her own symptoms as well as those of the child. Several factors might independently contribute to the child's increased awareness of internal feelings: actual illness that is reinforced by being kept home from school; greater maternal dissatisfaction and concern accompanied by both psychological and physical symptoms; and maternal attention to the child's symptoms. While no one factor may be important in itself, all of these variables occurring within the same family context may create a climate conducive to learning to focus on bodily concerns.

Response Bias

The analysis of predictors of psychological symptoms must be sensitive to biases in reporting such symptoms. There is a substantial literature dealing with response bias on measures of psychological symptoms,[28,29] particularly in respect to the social desirability response.[1] In the follow-up a four-item social desirability scale adapted from Crowne and Marlowe[30] ($\alpha = .52$) was included, as well as a six-item scale measuring the extent to which the respondent talks to others and complains about symptoms ($\alpha = .58$). Although this latter variable might reasonably be seen as an aspect of the distress reaction, a conservative approach was taken in which this scale is also treated as a measure of response bias. At the zero-order level, distress was correlated negatively with social desirability response ($-.16$) and positively with the tendency to complain ($.20$). When these two variables are taken into account, as shown in model 2 of the Table, they slightly enhance the predictability of the 1961 predictors.

As noted at the outset, reports of distress were not sex linked in this young sample in contrast to many other community populations.[31] Interpreting the absence of such a difference after the fact is an uncertain endeavor. It is conceivable that this sample of young adults who grew up during a period of social turmoil and changing sex role conceptions and expectations during the 1960s has been less influenced by socialization experiences differentiating the sexes in the expression of distress. Some data we have do not support such a view, however. For example, if socialization had changed fundamentally, we would anticipate no differences in the effects of social desirability on distress reports among men and women. Social desirability response, however, is significantly related to distress reports among men ($r = .27$) but not among women ($r = -.06$), suggesting that acknowledging distress symptoms is more stigmatizing for men.

Parental Influences on Reports of Adult Distress

Children with more illness, I have suggested, learn to attend to their internal states but do not differentiate between many physical and psychological feeling states. At early ages children define being healthy as feeling good, being able to do wanted things, and being happy. Feeling unhealthy, in contrast, is associated with not being able to engage in desired activities, feeling moody, and feeling weak.[32] Similarly, mothers in identifying illness in their children depend on behavioral signs. Change in the child's activity level is a central cue, and the most frequently noted indicators of illness are irritability, listlessness, apathy, crankiness, and the like.[33] One would presume that mothers differ in their attention to such cues, in their ability to identify illness in their children, and in their own reactions, and that their moods and feelings may influence the way they respond.[19] Thus mothers' responses may create varying degrees of reinforcement for children to monitor internal feelings as well as provide definitions for attributing meaning to internal states.

In the 1961 interviews with mothers we obtained some descriptive information on the way they would respond to their children's illnesses and their propensities to medicate them when ill, keep them home from school, and take them to doctors. These descriptions based on hypothetical items obtained in 1961 were not correlated to any appreciable degree with the level of psychological distress in young adulthood. Actual school absence, in contrast, was associated with distress.

In 1977 we obtained retrospective reports on a large number of parental behaviors and feelings about parents. Many of these retrospective reports were substantially associated with psychological distress, particularly measures of parental negative behavior—such as yelling or shouting at the child or insulting the child. The difficulty in interpreting these measures is that such reports may be distorted and may reflect the psychological state of the respondent more than actual parental behavior. Underlying the concern with parental behavior was the idea suggested by a variety of longitudinal studies that abuse and indifference of parents often linked with parental deviant behavior are associated with low self-evaluation, distress, and a variety of behavior disorders.[34–36] It was plausible that parental abuse and indifference, if it existed, would affect the child's tendency to monitor feelings, engage in self-assessment, and generally attempt to account for parental negative responses. Experimental work suggests that objective self-awareness most commonly results in negative evaluation,[37] and we might hypothesize that negative responses from parents would result in more self-appraisal and self-monitoring than in families in which the child feels accepted and loved. Indeed, both rejection itself and increased self-awareness may contribute independently to adult distress.

The available data do not allow one to place confidence in parental measures or to sort out alternative conceptions of family dynamics, but one intriguing finding suggests some interesting possibilities. In an earlier epidemiological study of college students, Greenley and Mechanic found that respondents high on a scale of identification with introspective others not only reported more psychological symptoms, but also were more likely to use medical, psychiatric, counseling, and other formal helping services.[38] In the present study, introspectiveness was measured by a scale in which respondents indicated the degree to which they were "sensitive and introspective," worried about meaning in life," and "interested in psychology" ($\alpha = .49$). Scores on this scale are correlated .47 with the distress measure despite the fact that the items do not directly measure symptoms and describe ordinary concerns. Moreover, when added to the regression equation it retains its strength as a predictor, overshadowing all other predictors (see model 3 of the Table). As one might anticipate, the introspectiveness score is related to parental variables similar to those predicting adult distress, particularly measures of parental negative behavior toward the child. It is conceivable that such a pattern of concern with self and self-scrutiny results when familial patterns are disrupted and such self-appraisal usually culminates in negative self-evaluation.[39] Introspection is also related to childhood symptoms and illness behavior, but these coefficients are statistically significant only in relation to school absence. In sum, a reasonable hypothesis to pursue is that persons who worry about meaning and the way they feel are more likely to focus on personal shortcomings and failures than others more oriented to the outer environment and task performance. Studies of astronauts—a group of high coping competence—for example, show great attention to the task environment and little psychological distress despite the dangers inherent in their missions.[40]

Comment

Predicting adulthood distress (itself a fluctuating state) on the basis of childhood factors is a "long shot." Moreover, such a global measure is a composite, reflecting a variety of causes including psychiatric disorder, learned patterns of illness behavior and response, and situational stress. Adulthood perception of stress and reports of parental negative behavior, for example, are related to symptom scores and contribute significantly to explaining variation in the regression analyses. Because these are all reports by the respondent at the same point in time, it can be argued that these reports and symptoms are varying aspects of the same underlying dimension, and thus these data have been deemphasized. Instead, the analysis focuses on the measures obtained in 1961 that predict distress in 1977 and thus eliminates such confounding.

Although adulthood distress is not comparable to psychiatric illness, persons with such diffuse complaints make major demands for medical, psychological, and social services. These patients are not well understood, are subjected to a wide variety of interventions, and are often a source of great frustration to physicians. Thus it is important to gain more understanding of the character of this "syndrome." The 1961 data are not sufficiently rich or detailed to depict reliably the complex dynamics of the way such syndromes initially develop, but they are consistent with the hypothesis that we are in part dealing with a learned pattern of illness behavior, with important developmental antecedents. Data have been presented that support the tentative conclusion that factors that focus the child's attention on internal states and that teach a pattern of internal monitoring contribute to a distress syndrome in adult life. The degree to which such a syndrome actually develops depends on the degree of psychological and bodily dysfunction, adverse life experiences, and other influences that reinforce a focus on internal feeling states. Independent experimental study has found that simply drawing a subject's attention to some aspect of bodily functions results in an increased prevalence of symptoms reported.[41]

The data presented here are consistent with the view that distress syndromes initially develop in childhood in families in which the mother is more upset and symptomatic, the child has more symptoms, and attention is directed to such symptoms by keeping the child home from school. Kerckhoff and Backs's suggestion that hysterical illness occurs among those under strain who do not know how to cope is a hypothesis worthy of further exploration.[25] Subsequent development of distress syndromes may represent some synthesis of bodily arousal, either endogenous or socially induced, learned patterns of attention or inattention to bodily experiences and feelings, and the interpretative schemas by which the person codes and copes with these. The data presented here take us only so far. Only through careful further developmental, experimental, and epidemiological research will we be able to assess the extent to which this working hypothesis is useful.

References

1. Dohrenwend BP, Dohrenwend BS: *Social Status and Psychological Disorder: A Causal Inquiry.* New York, John Wiley & Sons Inc 1969.
2. Dohrenwend BP, Dohrenwend BS: Social and cultural influences on psychopathology. *Ann Rev Psychol* 25:417–452, 1974.
3. Star SA: Psychoneurotic symptoms in the Army, in Stouffer SA, Guttman L, Suchman EA, et al (eds): *Studies in Social Psychology in World War II. The American Soldier: Combat and Its Aftermath.* Princeton, NJ, Princeton University Press, 1949, pp 411–455.
4. Langner T S: A 22-item screening score of psychiatric symptoms indicating impairment. *J Health Human Behav* 3:269–276, 1962.
5. Gurin G, Veroff J, Feld S: *Americans View Their Mental Health.* New York, Basic Books, 1960.
6. MacMillan AM: The health opinion survey: Techniques for estimating prevalence of psychoneurotic and related types of disorder in communities. *Psychol Rep* 3:325–329, 1957.

7. Brodman K, et al: The Cornell medical index—health questionnaire III: The evaluation of emotional disturbance. *J Clin Psychol* 8:119–124, 1952.

8. Dohrenwend BP: Some issues in the definition and measurement of psychiatric disorders in general populations, in the *Proceedings of the 14th National Meeting of the Public Health Conference on Records and Statistics*. Washington, DC, Government Printing Office, 1973, pp 480–489.

9. Mechanic D, Greenley JR: The prevalence of psychological distress and help-seeking in a college student population. *Soc Psychiatry* 11:1–14, 1976.

10. Schwartz CC, Myers JK, Astrachan, BM: Comparing three measures of mental status: A note on the validity of estimates of psychological disorder in the community. *J. Health Soc Behav* 14:265–273, 1973.

11. Weissman MM, Myers JK, Harding PS: Psychiatric disorders in a United States urban community: 1975–1976. *Am J Psychiatry* 135:459–462, 1978.

12. Frank J: *Persuasion and Healing: A Comparative Study of Psychotherapy*, rev ed. New York, Schocken Books, 1974.

13. *Report to the President From the President's Commission on Mental Health, 1978*. Washington, DC, Government Printing Office, 1978.

14. Mechanic D: The concept of illness behavior. *J Chron Dis* 15:189–194, 1962.

15. Mechanic D: Social psychologic factors affecting the presentation of bodily complaints. *N Engl J Med* 286:1132–1139, 1972.

16. Frank G: The role of the family in the development of psychopathology. *Psychol Bull* 64:191–205, 1965.

17. Sewell WH: Infant training and the personality of the child. *Am J Sociology* 58:150–159, 1952.

18. Marks IM: Research in neurosis: A selective view: I. Causes and courses. *Psychol Med* 3:436–454, 1973.

19. Mechanic D: The influence of mothers on their children's health attitudes and behavior. *Pediatrics* 33:444–453, 1964.

20. Mechanic D, Newton, M: Some problems in the analysis of morbidity data. *J Chron Dis* 18:569–580, 1965.

21. Mechanic D: *Medical Sociology: A Selective view*. New York, Free Press, 1968, pp. 159–166.

22. Wheaton B: The sociogenesis of psychological disorder. Reexamining the causal issues with logitudinal data. *Am Soc Rev* 43:383–403, 1978.

23. Tessler R, Mechanic, D: Psychological distress and perceived health status. *J Health Soc Behav* 19:254–262, 1978.

24. Ware JE, Jr, Davies-Avery, A, Donald, C: *Conceptualization and Measurement of Health for Adults in the Health Insurance Study: General Health Perceptions*. Santa Monica, Rand Report R-19871 5-HEW, September 1978, vol 5.

25. Kerckhoff AC, Back KW: *The June Bug: A Study of Hysterical Contagion*. New York, Appleton-Century-Crofts, 1968.

26. Lewis CE, Lewis MA, Lorimer A, et al: *Child Initiated Care: A Study of the Determinants of the Illness Behavior of Children*. Los Angeles, Final Report HS00773, Health Services Research Center, University of California, Los Angeles, August 1974 (PB-253-726/4WW).

27. Shepherd M, Oppenheim, AN, Mitchell S: Childhood behavior disorders and the child guidance clinic: An epidemiological study. *J Child Psychol Psychiatry* 7:39–52, 1966.

28. Seiler L: The 22-item scale used in field studies of mental illness: A question of method, a question of substance, and a question of theory. *J Health Soc Behav* 14:252–264, 1973.

29. Phillips D, Clancy K: Response biases in field studies of mental illness. *Am Sociol Rev* 35:503–515, 1970.

30. Crowne DP, Marlowe D: *The Approval Motive: Studies in Evaluative Dependence*. New York, John Wiley & Sons Inc, 1964.

31. Mechanic D: Sex, illness, illness behavior, and the use of health services. *J Human Stress* 2:29–40, 1976.

32. Natapoff J: Children's views of health: A developmental study. *Am J Public Health* 68:995–1000, 1978.

33. Mechanic D: Religion, religiosity, and illness behavior: The special case of the Jews. *Human Organization* 22:202–208, 1963.

34. Robins L: Follow-up studies of behavior disorders in children, in Quay H, Werry J (eds): *Psychopathological Disorders of Childhood*, ed 2. New York, John Wiley & Sons Inc, 1979.

35. Robins L: Longitudinal methods in the study of normal and pathological development, in Kisker KP et al (eds): *Psychiatrie der Gegenwart*, ed 2. Heidelberg, West Germany, Springer-Verlag, 1978, vol 1.

36. McCord W, McCord J, Gudeman J: *Origins of Alcoholism*. Palo Alto, Calif, Stanford University Press, 1960.

37. Duval S, Wicklund RA: *A Theory of Objective Self-awareness*. New York, Academic Press Inc, 1972.

38. Greenley JR, Mechanic D: Social selection in seeking help for psychological problems. *J Health Soc Behav* 17:249–262, 1976.

39. Wicklund R: Objective self-awareness, in Berkowitz L (ed), *Advances in Experimental Social Psychology*. New York, Academic Press Inc, 1975, vol 8.

40. Ruff G, Korchin S: Psychological responses of the Mercury astronauts to stress, in Grosser, G, et al (eds): *The Threat of Impending Disaster*. Cambridge, Mass, MIT Press, 1964.

41. Pennebaker JW, Skelton JA: Psychological parameters of physical symptoms. *Personality and Social Psychology Bulletin*, 1978, vol 4, pp 524–530.

11

Some Factors Associated with the Report and Evaluation of Back Pain

David Mechanic with Ronald J. Angel

Musculoskeletal problems are extremely prevalent and are responsible for much personal distress, absence from work, reduction of usual activities and use of medical and other types of professional care (Social Security Administration 1980). Data from the National Ambulatory Medical Care Survey (National Center for Health Statistics 1986) show back pain to be the most frequent pain complaint motivating a chronic pain visit (17.8 percent). Chronic back problems are also a major cause of permanent work disability in all nations. Such complaints constitute one of the largest components of problematic cases for evaluation faced by the Social Security Administration in administering the disability insurance system and by state agencies in administering workers' compensation.

Given the importance of chronic back pain to work disability, medical care costs, and government entitlement programs, and the magnitude of misery involved, it is remarkable how little we know about the epidemiology and natural history of these conditions (Nagi, Riley, and Newby 1973; Osterweis, Kleinman, and Mechanic 1987). This area is contentious, with common allegations of individuals malingering or being motivated by secondary gain, but there is relatively little systematic research devoted to the process of chronic pain and how it is affected by characteristics of individuals and their social settings over time. Least common are studies that systematically compare pain complaints of populations in relation to medical and disability evaluations, although there are some exemplary exceptions (Nagi 1969).

Survey data on back problems are difficult to evaluate because of variation in populations studied, the questions asked, the criteria used, the length of recall periods, and the uncertain relationship to disability. The Nuprin Pain Study (Harris and Associates 1985), a recent effort to make population estimates, reported that 56 percent of a national sample had backaches for one or more days, but only 15 percent had such pain for more than 30 days. These more frequent complaints were associated with increased age (50 or older), being female, not having completed high school, lower income, and other psychosocial characteristics.

Approximately four percent of the population reported that they had such severe back pain that they couldn't work or engage in routine activities for more than 30 days, and approximately two percent estimated such disability for 101 days or more. These estimates seem high compared with the National Health Interview Survey and other studies (Spitzer and Thomson 1986), but discrepant estimates could be explained by the vast differences in question format, recall periods, and samples used in these varying surveys. The surveys agree that back pain itself is very common, as is some related limited temporary disability, but only a very small subset of this larger group have long-term persistent disability. Spitzer and Task Force (1986), in a Canadian study, found that less than eight percent of patients complaining of back pain not supported by objective findings became chronic. A small percent of a large population, however, can account for a disproportionate amount of work absenteeism, use of medical resources, and demands on the disability insurance system. In Quebec, the 7.4 percent of spinal disorders involving more than six months lost from work accounted for more than 70 percent of the costs (Spitzer and Task Force 1986).

The dilemma, as noted earlier, concerns how much credibility to give to subjective complaints of pain and reports of inability to meet usual responsibilities when such claims have economic and other advantages. Since there are no definitve medical means to evaluate such claims (Chapman, Casey, Dubner, Foley, Gracely, and Reading 1985), except at the very extremes, it becomes especially important to understand as best we can what factors influence complaints and their evaluation. This paper makes a modest effort toward that end by examining data from the U.S. Health and Nutrition Examination Survey I (HANES).

Conceptual Approach: Pain and Illness Behavior

Pain is a subjective experience impossible to verify through objective medical assessment (Melzack 1973). Despite thorough medical evaluation, in many instances the persistence of subjective pain cannot be explained, although it may be apparent to the clinician that the patient is suffering great discomfort. The failure to verify subjective pain experience may reflect the inadequacy of medical concepts of pain and existing biomedical technology; conversely, it may reflect characteristics of individuals and their social contexts that influence the augmentation or suppression of pain experience.

It has long been observed that the social context and psychosocial need affect the individual's construction of pain, making it difficult to generalize from studies of laboratory pain. Much research demonstrates that pain has an important subjective component, and that there is no clear relationship between the amount of tissue damage and the degree of discomfort reported (Beecher 1959; Melzack 1973). In a classic observation, Beecher (1959) questioned wounded soldiers and a group of male civilians undergoing major surgery about their need for pain medication. While only one-third of the soldiers wanted medication to relieve their pain, 80 percent of the civilians wanted pain relief despite the fact that they were suffering from much less tissue trauma. Beecher interpreted these results in terms of secondary consequences: the soldiers' wounds were an escape from battle and the possibility of being killed, while to the civilian, surgical pain was viewed as a depressing, calamitous event which interfered with life goals. A classic sociological study by Zborowski (1952), demonstrating the important influence of cultural attitudes on pain reporting, focused largely on patients with disc disease and back pain. Subsequently, an enormous literature has developed on pain experience: its neurological and physiological bases; its perception, expression, and special language; its measurement; its management; and its link to social and cultural influences (Wall and Melzack 1984; Chapman et al. 1985; Fienberg, Loftus, and Tanur 1985; Keefe, Brown, Scott, and Ziesat 1982; Melzack 1983; Bonica 1980; Kleinman 1986; Osterweis, Kleinman, and Mechanic 1987).

In this paper, we examine two factors that appear to affect the evaluation of pain in the context of normal life situations: age and depressed mood. Many studies have found that elderly respondents report more positive health status relative to physician assessment or expected morbidity patterns (Maddox and Douglas 1973; Linn and Linn 1980; Friedsam and Martin 1963; Cockerham, Sharp, and Wilcox 1983), although there are occasional failures to replicate this finding (Levkoff, Cleary, and Wetle 1987). A number of researchers have suggested that elderly persons are health optimists, but such interpretation simply restates the finding without illuminating the process. A more viable suggestion is that the elderly adjust their perceptions because of modified health expectations with age (Tornstam 1975). The precise process is difficult to capture with survey data, but it is plausible to anticipate that assessments of pain are shaped by context, what people expect of themselves, and the consequences of pain for the roles and tasks they must assume, an observation commonly made in illness-behavior studies (cf. Mechanic 1978, pp. 249–89 and Mechanic 1986). Thus, we anticipate that elderly patients would be less likely than their younger counterparts to complain of back pain relative to objective measures.

Studies of illness behavior also find that negative health assessments are associated with depression, and that adverse psychological states affect self-perceptions and service utilization (Mechanic 1978; Tessler and Mechanic 1978; Blumer and Heilbronn 1982). There are alternative processes that might account for this association. Studies of pain and other distress states indicate that distraction reduces pain perception (Melzack 1973) and focus on the painful stimulus exacerbates discomfort (Mechanic 1983). Thus, it seems plausible that depression should augment chronic pain perception. In cross-sectional data sets, however, it is impossible to disentangle augmentation processes from the effects of pain and impairment on affective states.

Processes of augmentation can occur in a variety of ways. Many studies show that persons who report higher levels of distress perceive their general health more negatively (Tessler and Mechanic 1978). Such distress may affect perceptions of physical health and pain because these subjective responses are cognitively processed taking into account the larger context of social well-being. Depending on the context, pain may be experienced as more or less central to successful function. Alternatively, as evaluations are made in the context of depression and other adverse feeling-states, confusions between physical sensations and mental states may occur (Mechanic 1978; Imboden, Canter, Cluff, and Trever 1959; Imboden, Canter, and Cluff 1961).

Although pain reports are more specific and focused than general health perceptions, we anticipate that they are subject to some of the same influences.

Sample

This analysis is based upon data from the augmentation component of the HANES conducted from 1971 to 1975 (National Center for Health Statistics 1977). The augmentation component consists of a probability sample of 6,913 adults between the ages of 25 and 74 who received a detailed physical examination designed to obtain information on the prevalence of various common physical and mental disorders. Within this sample, the 2,431 persons (35 percent) who responded positively to one or more of five questions designed to identify symptoms of arthritis were then administered a supplemental questionnaire covering their functional capacities, pain experiences, medication, and appliance use. Thirty-nine percent of these respondents (937) reported having experienced pain in the back or neck for a month or more some time within the previous year. This subgroup, constituting 14 percent of the base sample, is the population that serves as the core of this analysis.

Measures

In order to identify factors mediating the experience of pain, we computed a summary score on the basis of the physical examination, termed "badback," which reflects the physician's evaluation of the extent of musculoskeletal symptomatology. In this examination the physician assesses the presence of scoliosis, kyphosis, lordosis, tenderness, limitation of motion, pain on motion, reflexion, extension, lateral bending, and rotation. A straight-leg-raising test is also done. We use as our measure the number of findings noted in this standardized examination. This measure has a range of 0–28 with a mean of 2.5 and a standard deviation of 3.4.

Responses from Supplement A of the survey, the arthritis self-report, of those reporting "pain in either the back or neck on most days for at least one month" are summed over seven additional questions. These questions ask whether the pain is present when resting; whether it awakens the respondent from sleep at night; whether it is made worse by coughing, sneezing, or deep breathing; whether it is made worse with bending or twisting motion; after prolonged activity; by prolonged sitting; or after prolonged standing. Scores on the resulting index, called "backcomplaint," range from 0–7 with a mean of 3.6 and a standard deviation of 2.0. This index is correlated .28 with the medical evaluation. Patients' complaints of back discomfort are much more frequent than physical findings that explain such complaints.

The data have limitations but reflect the common clinical situation wherein the patient complains of pain and disability and the physician attempts to assess to what degree physical findings can account for these complaints. It is worth noting that the standard physical exam used in HANES is comparable and probably superior to that found in typical outpatient medical practice. Comparison of our two measures serves as a crude indicator of the extent to which back and neck pain complaints are supported by physical findings.

In the clinical pain literature, there is continuing suggestion that psychological distress as measured by depressed mood and other states of dysphoria amplify pain complaints and contribute to their chronicity. (Blumer and Heilbronn 1982). Most data come from small clinical studies or cross-sectional surveys and cannot differentiate whether distress has causal significance or whether it results from persistent pain, or both. Unfortunately, HANES does not provide prospective observations on the individuals examined but it does allow examination of the distress pain association within a larger, more carefully studied sample.

Included in the HANES is a general well-being scale. This scale includes several items that measure depressed mood during the previous month: questions on feelings in general with responses ranging from "in excellent spirits" to "very low spirits"; a question on feeling "so sad, discouraged, hopeless, or had so many problems that you wondered if anything was worthwhile"; having felt down hearted and blue; and a ten-point rating scale on "how depressed or cheerful you have been." These items are comparable to those typically used in survey measures of depressed mood. Combining the items results in a scale with adequate reliability (alpha = .79).

Results

Table 11.1 reports the associations among measures used in our analysis. It shows that depressed mood is associated significantly with both back complaints (.16) and medically evaluated physical signs (.13). This suggests that whatever role depressed mood has, it is not solely a matter of self-perception. Depressed mood can, of course, affect both patients' responses in the clinical examination and how the doctor assesses these responses. The HANES data cannot speak to causal questions. Consistent with most epidemiological studies (Dohrenwend 1980; Myers, Weissman, Tischler, Holzer, Leaf, Orvaschel, Anthony, Boyd, Burke, Kramer, and Stoltzman 1984), depressed mood is significantly higher among persons with less education, those with lower incomes, women, blacks, unemployed persons, and those not married.

The relationship between age and our two measures of pain is particularly intriguing. Older respondents are more likely to be evaluated as having physical signs (.14) but age is negatively associated with back complaints (−.07), supporting the common belief that pain perceptions are dependent on context and social comparisons, an issue to which we will return.

Table 11.2, which presents sociodemographic characteristics associated with physician evaluations, amplifies the picture. Only 23 percent of pain patients evaluated have two or more physical findings. Those aged 56 or older are more than two times as likely to have such physical findings compared with the age groups 25 to 45, and approximately three times as likely to have five or more such findings. Similarly, those with some

TABLE 11.1
Associations Among Variables Studied (Pearson r) (N = 937)[1]

	Bad Back	Back Complaint	Depressed Mood	Age	Educ.	Low Income	Female	Black	Empl.	Married
Back Complaint	.283**									
Depressed Mood	.126**	.156**								
Age	.141**	−.070*	−.047							
Education	−.118**	−.061*	−.221**	−.299**						
Low Income[a]	.030	.050	.103**	.143**	−.300**					
Female	−.015	.064*	.120**	−.002	.056*	.017				
Black	.006	−.010	.154**	.035	−.272**	.127**	−.046			
Employed[b]	−.128**	−.036	−.110**	−.304**	.246**	−.156**	−.301**	−.047		
Married[c]	.011	.007	−.121**	.088**	.120**	−.197**	−.168**	−.098**	.050	

*Significant at <.05.
**Significant at <.01.

[1]Low income, female, black, employed, and married are dichotomous variables coded zero or one. The category listed in the table is coded one such that the coefficients refer to the impact of membership in the category. When one variable in a correlation is a dichotomy, the coefficient is a point biserial r, which indicates the impact on the continuous variable of membership in the relevant category of the dichotomy. When both variables are dichotomies, the coefficient is a Phi coefficient, interpreted in the same way as a Pearson correlation coefficient (Cohen and Cohen 1983).

[a]Dichotomous variable referring to total family income: 1 = less than $15,000; 0 = greater than $15,000.

[b]Refers to main activity during the past three months: 1 = working; 0 = keeping house or something else.

[c]1 = married; 0 = widowed, never married, divorced, separated.

TABLE 11.2
Relation of Back Exam Findings to Sociodemographic Characteristics
(Effective range of exam score 0–28; N = 2,431)

	Back Exam[1]						p[2]
	None	1	2	3	4	5	
Race							
White	23.3	54.2	6.1	4.1	3.3	8.9	NS
Black	20.8	54.3	7.6	5.0	2.2	10.1	
Age							
25–35	25.8	60.6	3.9	4.5	2.4	2.7	.00
36–45	29.1	57.4	2.8	3.3	2.3	5.1	
46–55	20.3	56.3	6.5	4.1	3.7	9.1	
56–64	21.0	50.2	8.2	3.9	3.4	13.3	
65 +	21.5	50.2	8.1	5.3	3.4	11.5	
Marital Status							
Married	22.3	55.4	6.1	4.1	3.4	8.7	NS
Nonmarried	24.7	51.2	6.8	4.6	2.5	10.3	
Income							
<$5,000	20.6	51.2	8.6	4.8	3.3	11.4	.00
$5,000–$9,999	22.2	54.7	5.6	4.7	3.6	9.2	
$10,000–$19,999	25.7	55.1	5.1	3.5	3.5	7.1	
$20,000 +	26.0	61.9	2.8	3.3	0.5	5.6	
Education							
High School or less	22.0	53.5	6.6	4.1	3.4	10.3	NS[3]
Some College +	26.4	57.7	4.9	4.9	1.6	4.5	
Depressed Mood							
High	19.2	42.4	8.8	5.6	5.6	18.4	.00
Low	23.1	55.0	6.2	4.2	3.0	8.6	
Sex							
Male	23.3	53.9	7.1	3.3	3.4	8.9	NS
Female	22.6	54.7	5.7	4.9	3.0	9.2	
Work Status							
Employed	26.8	56.6	5.0	3.6	2.6	5.3	.00
Other than Employed	19.4	52.3	7.4	4.8	3.7	12.5	
N	(556)	(1321)	(153)	(103)	(77)	(221)	
	(22.9%)	54.3%)	(6.3%)	(4.2%)	(3.2%)	(9.1%)	

[1]Number of physician findings.

[2]Based on chi-square tests.

[3]The difference between the two levels of education and the probability of having five or more physical findings is statistically significant at <.01.

college education and incomes in excess of $20,000 are less likely to have multiple physical findings, although the latter are not of statistical significance. Those with depressed mood are more than twice as likely to have five or more findings in contrast to those with more positive mood states. Finally, those with multiple findings are less likely to be employed.

In Table 11.3, the same sociodemographic characteristics are examined in relation to back complaints. In contrast to the data on physical findings, those aged 65 or older are least likely to complain, while those 46–55 are most likely to complain. Consistent with physical findings, those with depressed mood complained more, and those earning in excess of $20,000 had fewer complaints. There was little advantage of college education in respect to complaining in contrast to the earlier noted relationship with physician findings. The other associations were not particularly noteworthy.

The data presented suggest an intriguing relationship between age and the discrepancy between back complaints and physicians' physical findings. To explore this relationship further, we regressed the self-reported score (backcomplaint) on age and the physician evaluation score (badback). In this and the next model, both scores are standardized so that each has a mean of zero and a standard deviation of one. Age is categorized into five age ranges 25–35, 36–45, 46–55, 56–64, and 65 and over. The youngest group serves as the reference category. A negative coefficient represents less pain.

Table 11.4 presents the impact of age on reported back pain. This model reveals a monotonic decrease in reported pain by age category from the youngest group to the oldest. The only statistically significant effect, however, is for the oldest age category. Controlling for the physician's assessment insures that this association is not merely a reflection of increasing pathology.

Since other sociodemographic and economic factors might account for this age effect on the discrepancy between evaluated health and reported pain, we performed a multivariate analysis in which reported pain (backcomplaint) was regressed on evaluated status (badback) and other sociodemographic and economic variables. In addition, we include our measure of depressed mood.

Table 11.5 presents the results of three regressions. The first column presents coefficients for the entire sample. Not surprisingly, greater evaluated pathology is associated with more reported pain. In addition to evaluated status, however, only age and depressed mood are statistically significant. Again, increasing age decreases reported pain complaints. A lower score on depressed mood also results in less reported pain.

To test for a possible interaction of age with depressed mood, we divided

TABLE 11.3
Relation of Reported Back Complaints to Sociodemographic Characteristics
(N = 2,431)

| | Back Complaints[1] | | |
	Low (0–2)	High (3 or more)	p[2]
White	70.3	29.7	NS
Black	70.1	29.9	
Age			
25–35	72.1	27.9	.00
36–45	70.4	29.6	
46–55	64.7	35.3	
56–64	69.6	30.4	
65 +	76.9	23.1	
Marital Status			
Married	69.8	30.2	NS
Nonmarried	71.9	28.1	
Income			
<$5,000	70.8	29.2	NS[3]
$5,000–$9,999	71.6	28.4	
$10,000–$19,999	67.2	32.8	
$20,000 +	76.3	23.7	
Education			
High School or Less	70.3	29.7	NS
Some College +	71.4	28.6	
Depressed Mood			
High	50.4	49.6	.00
Low	71.4	28.6	
Sex			
Male	72.3	27.7	NS
Female	68.7	31.3	
Work Status			
Employed	71.9	28.1	NS
Other than Employed	68.8	31.2	
N	(1709)	(722)	
	70.3%	29.7%	

[1]Percentages add to 100% across (row percentages).
[2]Based on chi-square tests.
[3]The difference between those in the highest income category and all others is statistically significant at <.05. With the Yates correction, P = .057.

TABLE 11.4
Regression of Back Complaints on Age and Physician's Examination Score

Age Category[1]	Coefficient	Beta	N
Age Category			
36–45 years	.049	.018	(142)
46–55	.033	.015	(269)
56–64	−.100	−.043	(224)
65 +	−.356**	−.141	(183)
Back Exam (Physician)	.284**	.284	
Constant	.077		
Adjusted R²	.091		
(Sample Size)	(937)		

[1]Reference category = 25–35 (N = 119).
**Significant at <.01.

TABLE 11.5
Regression of Back Complaints on Physician Findings and Sociodemographic
Variables (standardized beta coefficients)

		Depressed Mood	
	Pooled	Low	High
Age	−.121**	−.184**a	−.048
Female	.060	.069	.081
Black	−.036	−.043	−.010
Married	.028	.078	−.024
Education	−.044	.039b	−.124**
Family Income			
$0,000–14,999	.051	.067	.049
$15,000–24,999	.004	−.002	−.002
Back Exam			
(Physician)	.284**	.207**b	.382**
Depressed Mood	−.099**	—	—
Adj. R²	.105	.064	.150
(Sample size)	(932)	(496)	(436)

**Significant at <.01.
aCoefficient significantly different from that of high depressed mood at <.01.
bCoefficient not significantly different from that of high depressed mood.

the sample of those high and low on depressed mood into approximate halves. Columns 2 and 3 of Table 11.5 present standardized beta coefficients for these two groupings. Again, as in the pooled sample, badback is a significant predictor of reported pain for both groups, although the size of the coefficient among the depressed respondents is almost twice as large as among the low depressed sample. The difference between the two coefficients (P = .08) fails to reach our established criterion for statistical significance. Among those who are more depressed, less education is also associated with more back complaints. In contrast, there is a significant age effect only for those in the low depressed mood category. The age coefficients for the two mood groups are significantly different (P < .01). These findings indicate, again, that evaluated physical findings affect back complaints for both high and low depressed mood groups but that older people with a greater sense of psychological well-being appear to complain less. The effect, although small, is statistically significant and comparable to the influence of physician findings.

It is possible, of course, that the experience of back pain is influenced by the presence of other conditions and that one's overall level of health may influence the association between tissue damage in any one location and the experience of pain at that same location. In order to test for such a possibility, we replicated the analyses presented in Tables 11.4 and 11.5, controlling for overall assessed health status.

Each respondent in our sample was examined by a physician who coded any conditions present according to International Classification of Disease (ICD) guidelines (U.S. Department of Health Education and Welfare 1967). In addition to recording the diagnosis, the physician rated the severity of each condition on a three-point scale as either minimum, moderate, or severe. We collapsed the individual ICD diagnoses into 12 broad categories and assigned respondents a score in each category, weighted by the physician's evaluation of the severity of the condition. Based on the ICD codes, the following categories were created: infectious diseases, cancers and neoplasms, metabolic disorders, blood diseases, diseases of the nervous system, circulatory diseases, respiratory diseases, digestive diseases, gastrointestinal disorders, skin conditions, diseases of the musculoskeletal system, and symptoms not elsewhere classified. Each respondent could have up to eight diagnoses. In order to control for overall health status, we employed this information in two ways. First, we entered a simple count of the number of diagnoses into the analyses presented in Tables 11.4 and 11.5. In addition, in order to take severity into account, we entered all 12 diagnostic categories, weighted by their respective severity scores, into the equations. In neither case did these controls significantly alter the associations.

Discussion

In this paper, we explored two lines of inquiry concerning the discrepancy between subjective back complaints and physician assessment. First, we found that older patients complained less of pain in comparison to other age groups than we would expect solely on the basis of physical findings. Subjective evaluations of health, we believe, are not absolute but, on the contrary, are made in a context of self and other comparisons, and are always relative to some degree. As people age, they may attribute some of their discomforts to the aging process and are more likely to normalize bodily discomforts. Moreover, they may feel that they are doing relatively well compared to their reference groups and the physical demands of their life regimen. Indeed, there may be less requirement for them to engage in the types of activities that exacerbate their discomforts.

These data are consistent with other studies of general health perceptions. Such perceptions are important because they are among the best general predictors of morbidity and use of medical care services (Ware 1986). Various studies find that such subjective assessments are significantly related to objective indicators such as physician assessments, medical record data, and longevity (LaRue, Bank, Jarvik, and Hetland 1979; Ferraro 1980; Fillenbaum 1979). Such measures also tend to reflect the influence of both physical and mental distress (Tessler and Mechanic 1978). Elderly individuals consistently report more positive health status than known patterns of morbidity or physician assessments would lead us to expect (Maddox and Douglas 1973; Linn and Linn 1980; Friedsam and Martin 1963; Cockerham et al. 1983).

We also found a relationship between depressed mood and the relative inclination to complain of back pain (controlling for physical findings). Moreover, the inclination of older persons to report less pain was not present among those with higher depressed mood, supporting our view that the psychological context of self-appraisal is crucial. We believe that psychological distress augments the experience of pain although our data also suggest that physical impairment may contribute to depressed mood. Clarification of such issues will require prospective studies and cannot be resolved by the types of data now available.

The finding in Table 11.5 that depressed patients with low education reported more pain was not anticipated, although many studies of low back pain and disability claimants suggest that education is an important predictive factor associated with such complaints. One explanation may be that persons with less education are in jobs, particularly unskilled labor, that involve tasks which exacerbate back pain. Also, persons with less education who are also depressed may be more alienated and have less coping facility, giving their pain greater centrality and significance in self-appraisals. These alternatives cannot be resolved using the types of secondary data reported here.

Finally, our findings suggest why clinicians have such difficulty in evaluating persistent pain complaints. Such complaints are highly complex responses reflecting not only sensations but the interpretations and evaluations that give them meaning in the context of the patient's life. These interpretations, and the illness conceptions on which they are based, help explain why persons with seemingly comparable physical status vary in their sense of distress and levels of incapacity. This is no way diminishes the reality of the complaint or its significance in the context of the individual's life and functioning.

References

Beecher, Henry Knowles. 1959. *Measurement of Subjective Responses: Quantitative Effects of Drugs*. New York: Oxford University Press.

Blumer, Dietrich, and Mary Heilbronn. 1982. "Chronic Pain as a Variant of Depressive Disease: The Pain-Prone Disorder." *Journal of Nervous and Mental Disease* 170:381–406.

Bonica, John J. (ed.). 1980. *Pain*. New York: Raven Press, pp. 143–54.

Chapman, C. R., K. L. Casey, R. Dubner, K. M. Foley, R. H. Gracely, and A. E. Reading. 1985. "Pain Measurement: An Overview." *Pain* 22:1–31.

Cockerham, William C., Kimberly Sharp, and Julie A. Wilcox. 1983. "Aging and Perceived Health Status." *Journal of Gerontology* 38:349–55.

Cohen, Jacob, and Patricia Cohen. 1983. *Applied Multiple Regression/Correlation Analysis for the Behavioral Sciences* (2nd ed.). Hillsdale: Lawrence Erlbaum Associates.

Dohrenwend, Bruce P. 1980. *Mental Illness in the United States: Epidemiological Estimates*. New York: Praeger.

Ferraro, Kenneth F. 1980. "Self-Ratings of Health among the Old and the Old-Old." *Journal of Health and Social Behavior* 21:377–83.

Fienberg, Stephen E., Elizabeth F. Loftus, and Judith M. Tanur. 1985. "Recalling Pain and Other Symptoms." *Milbank Memorial Fund Quarterly* 63:582–97.

Fillenbaum, Gerda G. 1979. "Social Context and Self-Assessments of Health among the Elderly." *Journal of Health and Social Behavior* 20:45–51.

Friedsam, Hiram, and Harry W. Martin. 1963. "A Comparison of Self and Physicians' Ratings in an Older Population." *Journal of Health and Social Behavior* 4:179–83.

Harris, Louis, and Associates. 1985. *The Nuprin Pain Report*. New York.

Imboden, John B., Arthur Canter, and Leighton E. Cluff, and Robert W. Trever, 1959. "Brucellosis III: Psychologic Aspects of Delayed Convalescence." *Archives of Internal Medicine* 103:406–14.

Imboden, John B., Arthur Canter, and Leighton E. Cluff, 1961. "Symptomatic Recovery from Medical Disorder." *Journal of the American Medical Association* 178:1182–84.

Keefe, Francis J., Charles Brown, Donald Scott, and Harold Ziesat. 1982. "Behavioral Assessment of Chronic Pain." Pp. 321–50 in *Assessment Strategies in Behavioral Medicine*, edited by F. J. Keefe, and J. A. Blumenthal. New York: Grune and Stratton.

Kleinman, Arthur. 1986. *Social Origins of Distress and Disease: Depression, Neurasthenia and Pain in Modern China*. New Haven: Yale University Press.

LaRue, Asenath, Lew Bank, Lissy Jarvik, and Monte Hetland. 1979. "Health in

Old Age: How Do Physicians' Ratings and Self-ratings Compare?'' *Journal of Gerontology* 34:687–91.

Levkoff, Sue, Paul D. Cleary, and Terrie Wetle. 1987. ''Differences in the Appraisal of Health Between Aged and Middle-Aged Adults.'' *Journal of Gerontology* 42:114–20.

Linn, Bernard S., and Margaret W. Linn. 1980. ''Objective and Self-Assessed Health in the Old and Very Old.'' *Social Science and Medicine* 14:311–15.

Maddox, George L., and Elizabeth B. Douglass. 1973. ''Self-Assessment of Health: A Longitudinal Study of Elderly Subjects.'' *Journal of Health and Social Behavior* 14:87–93.

Mechanic, David. 1978. *Medical Sociology*. (2nd ed.). New York: Free Press.

————. 1983. ''Adolescent Health and Illness Behavior. Review of the Literature and a New Hypothesis for the Study of Stress.'' *Journal of Human Stress* 9:4–13.

————. 1986. ''The Concept of Illness Behavior: Culture, Situation and Personal Predisposition.'' *Psychological Medicine*. 16:1–7.

Melzack, Ronald. 1973. *The Puzzle of Pain*. New York: Basic Books.

Melzack, Ronald. (ed.). 1983. *Pain Measurement and Assessment*. New York: Raven Press.

Myers, Jerome K., Myrna Weissman, Gary L. Tischler, Charles E. Holzer III, Philip J. Leaf, Helen Orvaschel, James C. Anthony, Jeffrey H. Boyd, Jack D. Burke, Jr., Morton Kramer, and Roger Stoltzman. 1984. ''Six-Month Prevalence of Psychiatric Disorders in Three Communities.'' *Archives of General Psychiatry* 41:959–67.

Nagi, Saad Z. 1969. *Disability and Rehabilitation: Legal, Clinical, and Self-Concepts and Measurement*. Columbus: Ohio State University Press.

Nagi, Saad Z., Lawrence E. Riley, and Larry G. Newby, 1973. ''A Social Epidemiology of Back Pain in a General Population.'' *Journal of Chronic Diseases* 26:769–79.

National Center for Health Statistics. 1977. *Plan and Operation of the Health and Nutrition Examination Survey, United States 1971–1973*. Series 1, No. 106, No. (HRA 77–1310). Rockville: Department of Health and Human Services.

————. 1986. ''The Management of Chronic Pain in Office-Based Ambulatory Care: National Ambulatory Medical Care Survey.'' *Advanced Data from Vital and Health Statistics*. No. 123. DHHS Pub. No. (PHS)86–1250.

Osterweis, Marian, Arthur Kleinman, and David Mechanic (eds.). 1987. ''Pain and Disability: Clinical, Behavioral and Policy Perspectives.'' Committee on Pain, Disability, and Chronic Illness Behavior. Institute of Medicine. Washington, D.C.: National Academy Press.

Social Security Administration, Office of Research and Statistics. 1980. *Work Disability in the United States: A Chartbook*. SSA Publication No. 13–11978.

Spitzer, Walter O., and Mary Ellen Thomson. 1986. ''Chronic Pain and Disability for Work.'' Paper prepared for the Committee on Pain, Disability and Illness Behavior. Washington: Institute of Medicine, National Academy of Sciences.

Spitzer, W. O., and Task Force. 1986. *Rapport du Groupe de Travail Quebecois sur les Aspects Cliniques des Affections Vertebrates Chez les Travailleurs*. L'Institute de Recherche en Sante et en Securite du Travail du Quebec.

Tessler, Richard C., and David Mechanic. 1978. ''Psychological Distress and Perceived Health Status.'' *Journal of Health and Social Behavior* 19:254–62.

Tornstam, Lars. 1975. ''Health and Self-Perception: A Systems Theoretical Approach.'' *The Gerontologist* 27:264–70.

United States Department of Health, Education and Welfare. 1967. *Eighth Revision International Classification of Diseases, Adopted for Use in the United States*. Washington, D.C.: U.S. Government Printing Office.

Wall, Patrick D., and Ronald Melzack. 1984. *Textbook of Pain*, New York: Churchill Livingstone.

Ware, John E., Jr. 1986. "The Assessment of Health Status." Pp. 204–28 in *Applications of Social Science to Clinical Medicine and Social Policy*, edited by L. H. Aiken and D. Mechanic. New Brunswick: Rutgers University Press.

Zborowski, Mark. 1952. "Cultural Components in Responses to Pain." *Journal of Social Issues* 4:16–30.

12

Distress Syndromes, Illness Behavior, Access to Care, and Medical Utilization in a Defined Population

David Mechanic, with Paul D. Cleary
and James R. Greenley

With growing interest in the relationship between general care and mental health,[1] attention has been refocused on the associations between psychiatric and physical morbidity and related help-seeking. From a policy perspective, there is interest in various studies suggesting that the provision of psychologic services reduces demands on the medical care system, and on the use of costly and possibly dangerous interventions.[2-3] Since the general medical sector is the major source of care for persons with psychologic problems and since such persons use a disproportionate amount of service, the indications that psychologic management of such persons reduces utilization are of major policy interest.

The literature on the relationship between psychologic morbidity and general medical utilization, however, is more uncertain than the results of such studies might indicate. All existing studies have major selection biases affecting which distressed persons receive psychologic management, making it difficult to interpret the significance of the utilization reduction. There is also a sizable literature on medical utilization indicating that patients receiving psychiatric treatment, as compared with those who do not, have higher levels of medical care utilization.[4-5] Given the importance of correct interpretation for policy decisions, as well as for understanding, we cannot simply dismiss the contradictions apparent in these two areas of literature.

The research literature referred to above supports the following general conclusions: 1) there is an association between reports of psychologic and physical distress, and persons with psychologic distress feel sicker and subjectively rate their physical health as less adequate[6]; 2) physical symptoms and psychologic distress both independently contribute to seeking general medical care[7]; 3) patients in psychiatric treatment use medical care of all kinds more frequently than those not receiving such care[4]; and 4) in some settings the provision of psychologic management is related to a reduction of medical utilization.[2]

These findings are amenable to alternative interpretations. The purpose of the present study was to examine in a defined population how patient status, distress, access to care and other variables are related to retrospective and prospective medical utilization (excluding psychiatric care).

The Research Setting

In 1977, we initiated a study of persons in north central Wisconsin who were served predominantly by a large multispecialty group practice and satellite clinics. Analyses presented here are based on two samples drawn from a defined area with a population of approximately 50,000:[1] 1) a representative sample of 1,026 persons 18 years of age or over in the population; and 2) a consecutive sample of 91 patients coming to the psychiatry department of the clinic for mental health services.[2] Eligibility for the second sample—referred to as the psychiatry sample—was based on four criteria: the patient had to 1) reside in the population area from which we drew our representative community sample; 2) be over 18 years of age; 3) have no record of consulting the psychiatric clinic in the previous 30 days; and 4) have a scheduled appointment of more than 15 minutes. The latter two criteria were used to define new episodes,[3] with the 15-minute criterion used to eliminate routine medication checks. We also excluded patients coming directly to obesity, smoking and alcoholism clinics administered by the psychiatric department. In both samples, respondents were interviewed in their homes and asked to complete a questionnaire and return it by mail following the interview. These data were then merged with retrospective and prospective data from respondents' medical and pharmacy records.

Measures of Psychologic Distress

Our data include a large number of scales of psychologic distress intended to measure varying types of psychopathology and expression patterns. In fact, these tend to be highly intercorrelated, and, thus, we focus on only six summary measures. The first, based on measures developed by Dohrenwend, which he calls *demoralization*,[8] is a summary score based on eight symptom scales most highly intercorrelated in Dohrenwend's PERI (Psychiatric Epidemiology Research Interview) questionnaire. The eight scales are self-esteem, hopelessness, dread, confused thinking, sadness, anxiety, psychophysiologic symptoms and perceived physical health. Scale construction followed Dohrenwend's procedures with slight modifications.

The second measure was a 22-item Langner scale.[9] The version used in this study was scored such that it had a range of 22 to 110[4] and in the representative sample had an internal consistency (coefficient Alpha) of 0.87. The third measure was a Distress Summary Score (I), based on 17 scales, most adapted from Dohrenwend, measuring drinking problems, psychophysiologic symptoms, problems that are possibly psychogenic, neurotic problems, obsessive symptoms, guilt, suicide-scale, enervation, anxiety, sadness, hopelessness and fears. Each scale was standardized, and these standardized scale scores were summated. A second Distress Summary Score (II) was constructed in a similar fashion, eliminating items from five scales (psychophysiologic, possible psychogenic, sleep problems, anxiety and enervation). The purpose of this fourth scale was to have a general psychologic distress indicator unconfounded by physical or psychophysiologic content. Two additional scales included in the analysis were the Eysenck Neuroticism Scale (coefficient Alpha = 0.55) and a Depression Scale composed of four previously mentioned scales (guilt, sadness, hopelessness and suicide). These six scales achieve adequate levels of reliability,[5] and have been found to be related to levels of functioning and illness behavior.

We examined the intercorrelations among these five measures for the cross-sectional and psychiatric samples (Table 12.1). These measures share many of the same items, and thus high intercorrelations are expected. With the exception of the Eysenck Neuroticism score, which is

TABLE 12.1
Correlations Between Distress Indicators
Psychiatric Sample (N = 91) Above Diagonal
Area Probability Sample (N = 1,026) Below Diagonal, Pairwise Deletion Used

	1	2	3	4	5	6
1. Demoralization	—	.93	.94	.86	.60	.81
2. Langner	.91	—	.89	.76	.63	.66
3. Distress summary I	.93	.90	—	.96	.60	.86
4. Distress summary II (psychologic)	.87	.80	.97	—	.55	.92
5. Eysenck	.58	.59	.56	.51	—	.45
6. Depression scale	.88	.78	.89	.90	.52	—

correlated 0.5 to 0.6 with the other measures, the remaining measures are very highly correlated in both the cross-sectional (0.8 to 0.9) and psychiatric (0.6 to 0.9) samples suggesting that it probably does not matter a great deal which is used. Eliminating anxiety, psychophysiologic concerns and physical symptom items from the distress summary score had little effect on how this score was correlated with other measures, and the two distress summary scores were correlated 0.97 in the sample of the general population and 0.96 in the psychiatric sample.

The samples were divided into the following groups: I—patients who came to the clinic for psychiatric care (the psychiatric sample); II—respondents in the cross-sectional sample whose medical records revealed a visit to a psychiatrist during the two-year interval in which we reviewed charts; III—those in the cross-sectional sample who had no record of psychiatric visits but who reported visiting a psychiatrist, psychologist, social worker or mental health center for a personal problem in the past year in the interview; and IV—those in the cross-sectional sample with no indication of mental health care. The treated samples had substantially higher scores on each of the six distress indicators, with the psychiatric sample scoring highest on each of the indicators (Table 12.2).[6]

Patient Status and Utilization

Medical records were examined for every medical provider named by respondents during the interviews, and we also examined the records of virtually all medical providers in the geographic area to ascertain whether our sample had used services without reporting such utilization. Patients who sought psychiatric care had higher levels of general medical utilization for both the retrospective and prospective periods (Table 12.3). For example, while nonusers of mental health services had visit rates of 2.6 and 2.4 medical visits for the retrospective and prospective periods, the rates for the psychiatric sample were 5.2 and 4.4 respectively. These differences were only slightly altered when adjusted for differences in age, sex and education among the samples.[7]

Unlike that in much of the existing literature, the definition of patient status in our study is independent of medical utilization and precedes the measurement of utilization in the case of the prospective data. While the results here are consistent with other studies, the reasons for these findings remain unclear. There are at least three major competing explanations: that medical utilization is a result of physical symptomatology concomitant with psychologic symptomatology; that use of both mental health and general medical services reflect generalized tendencies to seek help or related illness behavior; and that rates of high use of both types of service

TABLE 12.2

Mean Scores of Four Groups on Indicators of Distress*

(Standard Deviations in Parentheses)

	Cross-Sectional Sample of Population (Excluding Users of Mental Health Services)	Cross-Sectional Respondents with Psychiatric Record	Cross-Sectional Respondents Who Reported Using Mental Health Services	Psychiatric Sample
	(N = 842)	(N = 42)	(N = 28)	(N = 91)
1. Langner score	81	88	88	95
	(9.6)	(11.1)	(11.1)	(13.4)
2. Depression scale	58	64	67	75
	(8.6)	(9.7)	(15.8)	(14.0)
3. Distress summary score I	−0.41	7.8	8.7	14.9
	(10.3)	(12.2)	(14.7)	(13.7)
4. Distress summary score II	−0.24	4.9	5.9	10.1
	(7.5)	(8.3)	(11.7)	(9.6)
5. Demoralization score mean	5.2	7.8	7.8	10.6
	(3.4)	(4.0)	(4.4)	(5.1)
6. Eysenck neuroticism score mean	1.9	2.7	2.8	3.1
	(1.4)	(1.4)	(1.8)	(1.6)

*For all scales, higher scores correspond to higher symptom levels.

TABLE 12.3
Mean Scores on Retrospective and Prospective Medical Care Utilization (Excluding Mental Health)
(Standard Deviations in Parentheses)

	Cross-Sectional Sample of Population (Excluding Users of Mental Health Services)	Cross-Sectional Respondents with Psychiatric Record	Cross-Sectional Respondents Who Reported Using Mental Health Services	Psychiatric Sample
	(N = 842)	(N = 42)	(N = 28)	(N = 91)
Retrospective				
Medical utilization mean visits for year prior to interview	2.6	3.3	4.0	5.2
(Standard deviation)	(3.5)	(3.9)	(3.5)	(5.1)
Per cent 3 or more medical visits	35	48	61	57
Prospective				
Medical utilization mean visits for year following interview	2.4	3.8	3.8	4.4
(Standard deviation)	(3.6)	(4.0)	(3.1)	(4.9)
Per cent 3 or more medical visits	31	55	57	58

reflect overall access to both as indicated by method of payment for service and the accessibility of care.

As the first step in exploring alternative explanations, we compared the psychiatric, the cross-sectional respondents receiving mental health care (i.e., reported using mental health services and/or had a psychiatric visit in record), and the cross-sectional sample members who did not receive mental health care with respect to five measures of physical functioning, five measures of help-seeking and six measures of access to medical care (Table 12.4). The physical measures included a two-item subjective assessment of physical condition, a scale of six psychophysiologic symptoms, a scale of nine physical symptoms that are possibly psychogenic, reported number of chronic health conditions, and a measure of bed and hospital disability.[8] Help-seeking measures included three hypothetical scales of tendency to consult physicians (in the case of physical symptoms, in the case of psychologic symptoms and total combined scores), the patient's report of the importance of physical checkups and the patient's acknowledgment that it is appropriate to talk to doctors about personal problems. Access-to-care measures included whether the patient was a member of the prepaid plan, whether the patient reported having a personal doctor, whether the patient could name a specific doctor, convenience in getting to the doctor, difficulty getting an appointment and the reported number of days to get an appointment. Each of the physical morbidity and help-seeking measures significantly differentiated the samples, with the psychiatric sample being highest on almost all measures and the cross-sectional respondents who received no mental health care being lowest. The only exception to this pattern was that reported mental health services users had the highest tendency to consult a physician for physical reasons and scored highest on the combined scale of tendency to consult physicians. There were no statistically significant differences among the samples in access to care.

Next, we examined the extent to which age, education and sex differences across the groups explained the utilization patterns. Only sex was a significant predictor of use, with women using more services. The unadjusted differences in medical utilization for one year between the psychiatric sample and the cross-sectional sample members who did not use mental health services was 2.6 visits in the retrospective period and two visits in the prospective period. In other words, the excess of medical visits in the psychiatric sample compared with the cross-sectional non-mental health help seekers was 100 per cent for retrospective data and 83 per cent for prospective data. Adjusting for sex differences among samples reduces the medical utilization differences to 2.3 visits for retrospective data and 1.8 visits for prospective data (Tables 12.5 and 12.6).[9]

TABLE 12.4

Means Scores on Measures Reflecting Alternative Hypotheses Accounting for Utilization Differences

	Cross-Sectional Sample		Psychiatric Sample
	Non-Mental Health Users	Mental Health Users	
	(N = 842)	(N = 70)	(N = 91)
Hypothesis 1—Physical Morbidity			
Perception of Physical Condition	5.1	5.5	5.6*
Psychophysiologic symptoms	20.5	21.6	22.8*
Possible psychogenic symptoms	29.1	30.6	31.3*
Number of chronic health conditions	2.6	3.4	3.7*
Bed and hospital disability	0.5	0.7	0.9*
Hypothesis 2—Help-Seeking Tendencies			
Tendency to consult doctor-total	4.3	5.1	4.2*
Tendency to consult doctor-psychologic	0.4	0.5	0.5*
Tendency to consult doctor-physical	4.0	4.6	3.7*
Thinks it important to have checkups	6.1	6.5	7.0*
Thinks it appropriate to talk to doctor about personal problems	2.5	2.8	3.0*
Hypothesis 3—Access to Care			
Proportion naming an individual doctor	0.6	0.7	0.6
Proportion in prepaid group	0.4	0.5	0.7
Has no personal doctor for overall health needs	1.5	1.3	1.4
Inconvenient to get to doctor	1.2	1.2	1.3
Days wait for appointment	23.0	22.3	17.8
Difficulty getting appointment	1.4	1.2	1.4

*One-way analysis of variance among the three groups significant at the 0.05 level.

TABLE 12.5
Medical Utilization Among Groups Controlling for Sex, Illness Behavior and Physical Symptoms

	Cross-Sectional Sample		Psychiatric Sample
	Non-Mental Health Users	Mental Health Users	
	(N = 842)	(N = 70)	(N = 91)
Unadjusted medical care utilization			
Retrospective	2.6	3.6	5.2
Prospective	2.4	3.8	4.4
Medical care utilization adjusted for sex			
Retrospective	2.6	3.5	4.9
Prospective	2.5	3.7	4.3
Medical care utilization adjusted for five physical symptom measures			
Retrospective	2.7	3.2	4.4
Prospective	2.5	3.5	4.0
Medical care utilization adjusted for illness behavior measures			
Retrospective	2.8	3.4	4.6
Prospective	2.6	3.6	4.3
Medical care utilization adjusted for sex and significant physical symptoms* and illness behavior measures			
Retrospective	2.9	3.3	4.2
Prospective	2.7	3.3	3.9

*In retrospective analysis, scale of "symptoms possibly psychogenic" was used; in prospective analysis, perceived physical status was used.

TABLE 12.6
Differences in Mean Medical Care Utilization Between Cross-Sectional Sample Who
Are Nonusers of Mental Health Services and Psychiatric Sample

	Retrospective	Prospective
Unadjusted difference	2.6	2.0
Adjusted by sex	2.3	1.8
Adjusted by physical measures	1.7	1.5
Adjusted by illness behavior measures	1.8	1.7
Adjusted by sex, physical measures and illness behavior	1.3	1.2

We suggested three hypotheses that may account for differences in utilization among these samples: the first explanation accounts for the differences on the basis of magnitude of physical symptoms accompanying psychologic disorder, the second on the basis of differential help-seeking tendencies and the third on the basis of access. Because there were no significant differences among the groups in access, we focused on the first two hypotheses. Thus, we separately adjusted medical utilization rates among the samples by the five physical and psychophysiologic illness scales that differentiated these groups and by the four illness behavior measures on which the groups varied. Controlling for the physical symptom measures reduces the difference of 2.6 visits for retrospective data and two visits for prospective data to 1.7 and 1.5 reductions of 35 per cent and 25 per cent, respectively. Controlling for illness behavior measures reduces the differences to 1.8 and 1.7 visits, reductions of 31 per cent and 15 per cent, respectively. Next, we constructed regression equations to correct utilization for the best combination of significant predictors. In the case of retrospective utilization, four variables—sex, a scale of physiologic symptoms that could be psychogenic, a measure of bed disability—hospital days, and a measure of the respondent's belief in having regular checkups even when feeling well—reduced group differences for retrospective data to 1.3 visits, a reduction of 50 per cent. Similarly, four predictors—sex, perceived health, bed disability-hospital days, and the respondent's belief in having regular checkups—reduced the prospective difference to 1.2 visits, a reduction of 40 per cent (Table 12.6).

Concomitant Physical and Psychologic Morbidity

The fact that reported physical morbidity is the best discriminator between users and nonusers of psychiatric facilities suggests that it is important to investigate the link between physical and psychologic morbidity. Our study was not designed to investigate this relationship, but by examining the types of physical conditions differentiating the two groups, we can better understand why physical morbidity is predictive of psychiatric use. There are at least four general hypotheses that can account for the association between physical and mental health: 1) certain people are constitutionally resistant or vulnerable to both physical and mental health problems; 2) psychologic distress may be an etiologic factor in certain physical diseases; 3) the effects of physical diseases may lead to or exacerbate the development of psychologic problems; or 4) particular persons may be more sensitive to or aware of both physical and mental states. To investigate the relative plausibility of these different explanations, we examined all the items included in the physical morbidity indices and examined which particular conditions best accounted for the higher distress scores among psychiatric users. With few exceptions, users of the psychiatric clinic were more likely than nonusers in the cross-sectional sample to report psychophysiologic and psychogenic symptoms. The only symptoms psychiatric clinic users did not report significantly more frequently were constipation, high blood pressure and asthma attacks. There was virtually no difference between the two groups in reported frequency of constipation (p = 0.47) or high blood pressure (p = 0.65), but the difference in reported frequency of asthma was in the expected direction and approached statistical significance (p = 0.08). Psychiatric clinic users were also more likely to report numerous ailments, poorer perceived health, and more bed and hospital disability. When chronic health conditions were examined, however, there were significant differences for only eight of the 27 conditions. Those reported significantly more frequently by the psychiatric patients were asthma, repeated attacks of sinus problems, stomach ulcer and other chronic stomach problems, allergies, prostate trouble or repeated urinary tract infections, tremor or shaking, and repeated troubles with back or spine.

These results are at best suggestive, but it is notable that with the exception of prostate trouble and repeated urinary tract infections, all the chronic conditions reported more frequently by patients in the psychiatric sample are conditions frequently viewed as having a psychogenic component. This is not true of most of the conditions for which the groups did not differ.

These findings are consistent with two of the hypotheses mentioned previously: that psychologic factors may be etiologic factors in certain diseases, and that certain persons may be more attentive to both their mental and physical condition. For all the chronic conditions more prevalent in the psychiatric sample, with the exception of prostate and urinary tract problems, one could reasonably argue that either 1) stress could lead to or exacerbate the problem, or 2) that it is the type of condition that would be more likely to be noticed and reported if a person was more sensitive and attentive to his/her physical state. On the other hand, none of the severely disabling conditions, such as stroke, arthritis, diabetes, cancer and paralysis, which might be expected to result in despair or depression, was significantly more prevalent among the users of the psychiatric clinic. It is becoming increasingly recognized that the linkage between physical and mental health is a complex and important one. Understanding the utilization patterns of persons with psychiatric problems will require careful analysis of the occurrence of symptoms.

Multivariate Analyses Within Samples

All of the analyses, thus far, have been confined to differences between groups. As part of our analysis, we also examined factors affecting utilization within the cross-sectional samples of mental health help-seekers and non-help seekers, and within the psychiatric sample. Because the mental health help-seeking samples are small, very few predictors achieve statistical significance, and the only factors we could identify within the psychiatric sample and the help-seeking cross-sectional sample that accounted for differences in medical utilization were measures of health perceptions and disability.

In the case of cross-sectional respondents who did not seek mental health services, significant predictors of use of medical care were access to care, illness behavior and physical symptoms. Whether the respondent is in a prepayment plan, can identify an individual personal doctor and reports little difficulty in getting an appointment help explain medical utilization. These three predictors account for 5 per cent of utilization in the retrospective data, and the first two predictors account for 2 per cent of utilization in the prospective data.

On the assumption that access to care enables people to use services who wish them (either because they have symptoms or particular illness behavior patterns), we entered the three access variables mentioned above as fixed predictors and then examined what combination of physical illness measures and illness behavior measures yielded the best predictors of variations in medical utilization. In the case of prior utilization, the access measures—reported bed-disability days and belief in the importance of regular checkups—accounted for 15 per cent of variation in utilization. The best predictor was reported bed-disability. We were less successful in predicting prospective medical utilization. Membership in a prepaid plan, identifying a personal physician, reported bed-disability days and subjective assessment of physical condition accounted for 6 per cent of variation in utilization (Table 12.7).

TABLE 12.7
Regression Models of Medical Care Utilization in the Cross-Sectional Sample

	Retrospective (beta)	Prospective (beta)
Model 1—Access		
Not in prepaid plan	−0.13*	−0.10*
Does not name a regular doctor	−0.13*	−0.08*
Difficulty getting an appointment	−0.09*	
R^2	0.05	0.02
Model 2—Access, Illness Behavior and Physical Symptoms		
Fixed variables		
Not in a prepaid plan	−0.11*	−0.09*
Does not name a regular doctor	−0.04	−0.05
Difficulty getting an appointment	−0.07	
Second step		
Bed-hospital days	0.29*	0.16*
Says regular checkups important	0.12*	
Poor subjective physical condition		0.12*
R^2	0.15	0.06

*$p < .05$.

As noted in the introduction, a central issue in the study of medical care use has been whether providing psychologic services reduces the utilization of other medical services by distressed patients. One hypothesis is that high utilization rates may reflect, in part, help seeking for psychologic problems, and if psychologic services are provided they will be "offset" by a corresponding reduction in medical care use. Although our data were not collected to address this issue, by comparing the utilization patterns of distressed patients who used the psychiatric clinic with those of patients in the population sample with comparable levels of distress, we can get some indication as to whether an offset has occurred among the users of the psychiatric clinic.

Because one would expect the impact of psychiatric services to be greatest for those patients who are most distressed, we analyzed utilization patterns among those patients with a demoralization score that was above the 90th percentile of the general population sample. Thus, the figures reported are based on 46 people from the sample of psychiatric clinic users and 76 people from the population sample who had demoralization scores above this criterion. Among these people, the change in utilization rates over the period of the study supports the offset hypothesis; the utilization of distressed people who did not use psychologic services increased from 3.04 visits per year (in the year prior to the interview) to 3.25 visits per year (in the year subsequent to the interview), while medical care use among distressed persons from the sample of psychiatric clinic users decreased from 5.54 visits per year to 4.57 visits per year. However, neither of these differences nor the contrast of these differences was statistically significant. In addition, there are several limitations of the data that must be kept in mind when interpreting these results. First, we have no way of determining if any of the medical care visits by people in the psychiatric sample were solely for the purpose of obtaining a referral to the psychiatric clinic. Thus, the decrease of less than one visit per year among psychiatric clinic users might partially be accounted for by a referral visit in the year preceding the interview. A second problem is one common to almost all studies addressing the offset question: the sample of psychiatric clinic users is a self-selected sample. Presumably, the persons who seek psychiatric care are most likely to do so at a time when their need for help is greatest. Consequently, one would expect that their use of nonpsychiatric services would also be highest preceding such a visit. Even if there were no treatment effects, one would expect some reduction of both distress and help-seeking behavior (both psychiatric and nonpsychiatric). In short, although there is some indication of an offset effect among patients receiving psychiatric care, this effect, even if free of methodologic ambiguities, would be trivial in comparison with the excess medical utilization of psychiatric patients as compared with patients who are not in psychiatric care.

Discussion

In short, we have been able to explain almost half of the differences in medical utilization among groups who are mental health care seekers and nonusers of mental health services. We have confirmed, using independent records and on a prospective basis, that users of mental health services also use substantially more general medical services. Such differences are in part due to physical symptoms and disorder concomitant with psychologic disorder and higher illness behavior propensities. Physical symptoms and disability appear to have more impact on utilization than differences in illness behavior.

A surprising finding in the cross-sectional sample was that psychologic distress as measured by various screening scales had only a very modest relationship to retrospective and prospective medical utilization. While such relationships are significant at the zero-order level, they are not significant when controls are introduced for access, physical symptoms and illness behavior. The weak impact of distress on utilization relative to some other studies may reflect the special characteristics of this rural population. The population studied appears to be a highly stoical, self-reliant group, many of Northern European and Scandinavian backgrounds. In the United States in 1977, there were 3.3 visits per person to a doctor's office, clinic or group practice, and 3.2 visits in the north central states and outside Standard Metropolitan Statistical Areas.[10] In contrast, our cross-sectional sample had 2.4 visits for the prospective period and 2.6 visits for the retrospective period. It is plausible that distress as a determinant of general medical services is more substantial in situations in which medical care is defined broadly and in which discretionary use is more consistent with cultural patterns in the population.

The data presented here are not consistent with a growing literature suggesting that psychiatric intervention among distressed persons results in reduced medical utilization. Persons receiving mental health services had considerably higher medical utilization for both the retrospective year and for the year following contact with psychiatric services. It is possible that medical utilization for these patients will show a reduction in subsequent years. There are many reasons to assist psychologically distressed persons. Whether reduction in medical utilization occurs has not been firmly established, and studies demonstrating this effect have significant methodologic limitations.

In sum, there are at least three general interpretations for the high rates of medical utilization among patients who receive psychiatric services: that the link is due to the interrelationships between psychologic symptoms and physical symptoms; that it reflects high generalized help-seeking propensities; and that it reflects broader access to both medical and psychiatric services. Although we find some evidence in support of each of these interpretations, the explanation that is most powerful is that high medical utilization among patients receiving mental health services is a product of physical symptoms and discomfort concomitant with psychologic disorder.

Notes

1. Because we did not use a simple random sample, in some cases our calculations may slightly overestimate the p-values of significance tests.
2. Psychiatric patients were concerned with confidentiality, and twenty-eight patients asked not to be included in the study. Because such a high refusal rate could bias our results, we compared our sample with those who did not participate in the study to see how they differed on a variety of dimensions. There were no significant differences between our sample and those who refused to participate in presenting diagnosis, number of visits to the psychiatry department over a two-year period, mean age, marital status or sex. These two groups did differ with respect to past psychiatric history. Eight per cent of our

sample had been hospitalized prior to the study for a psychiatric problem in contrast to 43 per cent of those who refused to participate. It appears that the patients we lost had either more severe or more chronic conditions than those included in the sample.

3. Twenty-three of the patients in our psychiatric sample had indications in their charts that they had sought psychiatric care at some time in the past. We examined how these patients differed from patients without prior episodes on 50 variables, and the only statistically significant difference was that those with a prior episode had slightly less education.

4. For each item in the Langner scale, respondents were asked whether they had experienced that symptom very often, fairly often, sometimes, almost never or never in the prior three months. The responses to these items, which were scored as 5, 4, 3, 2 or 1, were then summed to form the Langner score.

5. The internal consistencies (coefficient Alpha) for the components of the various summary measures are: self-esteem (0.72), hopelessness (0.78), dread/fear (0.43), confused thinking (0.79), sadness (0.81), anxiety (0.82), psychophysiologic symptoms (0.52), perceived physical health (0.45), drinking problems (0.77), manic behavior (0.56), delusions (0.52), explosiveness (0.72), sleep problems (0.63), possible psychogenic problems (0.60), neurotic problems (0.69), obsessive symptoms (0.70), guilt (0.75), suicide-scale (0.73), enervation (0.75).

6. Utilization data, of course, were obtained only for respondents who gave legal consent for such access (89 per cent of the cross-sectional sample). To simplify comparisons, all subsequent analyses are based only on the respondents for whom we have medical record data. Those who did not consent to have their records reviewed were compared with those who did and were found to be slightly older, less educated and with lower incomes than those who gave consent. In addition, they were lower on some of the measures of psychologic distress; were less likely to be involved in clubs and social activities; and were less likely to respond that they trusted their physician, that they felt comfortable in discussing emotional problems with him or that they had friends who had used a psychiatrist. In general, the differences were relatively small and are not likely to greatly influence inferences made from the data because of the high response rate.

7. Although our analyses focuses on use of outpatient services, people in the psychiatric sample were also likely to be hospitalized. Nonusers of mental health services had an average of 0.10 and 0.11 hospital admissions for the retrospective and prospective periods, while the rates for the psychiatric sample were 0.23 and 0.15, respectively.

8. The psychophysiologic symptoms asked about were: poor appetite, constipation, headaches, cold sweats, trembling hands and acid stomach. The possible psychogenic symptoms were: dizziness, fainting spells, heart beating hard, chest pains, shortness of breath, high blood pressure, asthma, diarrhea and weight change without being on a diet. The chronic conditions asked about were: asthma, chronic bronchitis, sinus trouble, rheumatic fever, hardening of the arteries, high blood pressure, heart trouble, stroke, varicose veins, hemorrhoids or piles, hay fever, gall bladder or liver trouble, stomach ulcer, stomach problems, kidney trouble, arthritis, diabetes, thyroid trouble or goiter, allergy, epilepsy, cancer, skin trouble, hernia or rupture, prostate or urinary problems, tremors, paralysis and chronic back problems.

9. All adjusted means were calculated using analysis of the covariance on the combined, unweighted groups. This procedure assumes that the relationship bètween the covariates and the dependent variables are the same in each group, an assumption difficult to test with such small groups.

References

1. President's Commission on Mental Health. Report to the President, Vol. I. Washington, D.C.: United States Government Printing Office, 1979.
2. Jones K, Vischi T. Impact of alcohol, drug abuse and mental health treatment on medical care utilization: a review of the research literature. Med Care 1979;17(Suppl.): entire issue.
3. Mumford E, Schlesinger H, Glass G. Problems of analyzing the cost offset of including a mental health component in primary care. In: Institute of Medicine. Mental Health Services in General Health Care. Washington, D.C.: National Academy of Sciences, 1979; 101.
4. Hankin J, Okay J. Mental disorder and primary medical care: an analytical review of the literature. Rockville, Maryland: National Institute of Mental Health Series.D, No. 5, 1979.
5. Eastwood M. The relation between physical and mental illness. Toronto: University of Toronto Press, 1975.
6. Tessler R, Mechanic D. Psychological distress and perceived health status. J Health Soc Behav 1978;19:254.
7. Tessler R, Mechanic D, Dimond M. The effect of psychological distress on physician utilization: a prospective study. J Health Soc Behav 1976;17:353.
8. Dohrenwend B, et al. Nonspecific psychological distress and other dimensions of psychopathology in the general population: measures for use in the general population. Arch Gen Psychiatry 1980;37:1129.
9. Langner T.S. A twenty-two item screening score of psychiatric symptoms indicating impairment. J Health Soc Behav 1962;3:269.
10. Office of Health Research, Statistics and Technology. Health, United States. Hyattsville, Maryland: Public Health Service, 1979. (DHEW Publication (PHS) 80–1232, p. 186.)

Part IV
CHALLENGES AND CHOICES IN HEALTH CARE ORGANIZATION

13

Alternatives to Mental Hospital Treatment: A Sociological Perspective

There has been an impressive growth of attention devoted to the management of psychotic disorders in the community as compared with hospital contexts. The encouragement for this emphasis has come from various quarters: changes in philosophical and administrative attitudes concerning the retention of the mentally ill in mental hospitals, altered funding patterns, and the growth of a vigorous civil liberties movement on behalf of the mentally ill (Golann and Fremouw, 1976). The development and refinement of drug therapy for psychotic conditions, which alleviated the most blatant and bizarre manifestations of the psychoses, gave the hospital, the community, and the families of the mentally ill increased confidence that this displacement of responsibility was feasible and productive (Mechanic, 1969). While this social movement was to some extent encouraged and supported by research on the rehabilitative process, the fact was and still remains that we have only the most crude understanding of the social forces in the community that help contain psychotic behavior and help maintain the psychotic at a reasonable level of social functioning.

While there have been an impressive number of community demonstrations of the feasibility of alternatives to hospitalization, and some evidence of atrocities when responsibility for maintaining an adequate system of services was not exercised, much of our experience has been gained through trial and error and not through any sophisticated theory of intervention. While a body of research did develop, documenting the erosive influences of custodial dependency and inactivity, much of our more positive evidence of the ability to successfully contain psychotic behavior in the community came from a large number of demonstration programs, carried out in different communities, that developed ad hoc explanations to account for the results achieved. Much of the research stems from the good sense and wisdom of clinicians concerned with community care rather than from any consistent theoretical framework or sophisticated understanding of basic processes.

As we look to the future, we would do well to strive more vigorously for a systematic perspective that more clearly poses the research and evaluation issues that must be dealt with if community care alternatives to hospitalization are to develop more focused and targeted interventions to deal with the great variety of problems that continue to persist. These problems are obvious at the level of individual functioning of the psychotic patient, at the level of the community and the social and social psychological processes affecting the provision of services and their outcomes, and at the more global social and political level as it affects the definitions and care of the mentally ill. I shall address each of these issues in turn.

Individual Functioning

At the level of individual functioning we still have a great deal to learn about the range of intervening variables that play an important part in the progression of mental illness. These intervening variables may characterize the person: his biological constitution, his individual capacities, his values, life orientations, and coping devices. Or they may be characteristic of the larger social environment as typified by the degree of stress, stimulation, or noxious agents to which he is exposed, the social assaults that characterize his life situation, and the network of social supports available to him. In thinking about problems of studying adaptation, I have found it useful to consider five types of deficiencies affecting the disruption of effective behavior. This classification may be a useful way to organize our thinking about the intervening variables that require more study, and they might possibly be useful in designing services for psychotic patients.

1. A major impediment to effective social functioning is the *lack of material resources* necessary to sustain the person or social group. While the link between poverty and illness is certainly not direct, the lack of material resources contributes to the problems of adaptation among vulnerable persons and increases the probability of disorganized behavior. Brenner (1973), for example, has found that economic recessions are followed by increased admissions to mental hospitals, and he makes a reasonable case that these correlations are not easily explained simply as a result of changing definitions of disorder under changing economic conditions.

At the most primitive level, the adequacy of nutrition and shelter is central. Inadequate nutrition, in particular, has been linked to a general vulnerability and increased mortality resulting from disease, and affects both social and intellectual development. In reference specifically to psychotic patients, there are continuing indications of gross deficiencies in the material environment necessary for a minimal standard of living quality. As communities have mounted political pressures to resist board and care facilities, halfway houses, and outpatient facilities, mental health departments have often followed the line of least resistance, locating such facilities in the most ecologically disorganized areas of the city. Patients in such areas suffer high risk of victimization and may further be exposed to the anomie and hopelessness that frequently pervade these environments.

2. *Lack of Appropriate Skills.* The adequacy of any social group or of individuals depends on the effectiveness of cultural preparation and the availability of problem-solving tools necessary to deal with their environments. What may be an ordinary situation to those with skills or otherwise adequate cultural preparation is a crisis for those who lack them. As care for psychotic patients has increasingly been provided in community contexts, it has become more apparent how frequently such patients lack basic skills essential for everyday living. While the problem of the psychoses extends well beyond inadequacies of skills and cultural preparation, the absence of these skills, or their erosion due to the chronic course of the illness, very much exacerbates the problems of such patients in the community. It makes it more difficult for them to find and maintain employment, to establish functional interpersonal relationships, to enjoy adequate living quarters, and to avoid difficulties with the authorities. Moreover, the dependency of the chronic psychotic patient means that these patients are likely to have continuing contacts with official bureaucracies, and skills in handling these become important for their satisfactory community adjustment. Some interesting efforts have been initiated to assist chronic schizophrenics in improving everyday skills on the assumption that these contribute not only to more adequate social functioning, but also help avoid repeated rehospitalizations. While the evidence is not all in, there are indications that this approach facilitates more effective community performance, at least in the short run.

Speaking more generally, there is a growing body of evidence suggesting that the movement of population from one environment to another, such as from rural to industrial life and from country to city, is associated with a higher prevalence of disease of a variety of kinds (Dubos, 1959). Perhaps the group least fitted for major social and cultural change, but subjected to it as a matter of course, are chronic psychotic patients who increasingly reside in unfamiliar settings with limited social supports. Although we still lack definite evidence to suggest that providing simple skills contributes to a more favorable course in the progression of pyschosis, it would seem prudent to give this area greater emphasis than at present.

3. *Lack of Adequate Defenses.* Man's ability to engage in effective behavior depends not only on constitution and past preparation, but also on psychological capacities to deal with signals of danger and hopelessness that hamper continued coping efforts. Cultural and personal devices must be available to the person to contain and control feelings that hamper long-term adaptations and to facilitate continued attention to ordinary activities rather than to flight. It is well established that schizophrenic patients have difficulties in dealing with intense personal relationships, for whatever reason, and patients with a vulnerability to depression appear to be unusually susceptible to situations in which they suffer a sense of loss.

Building stronger personal defenses is perhaps the most difficult aspect of improving adaptation, yet this is the area where traditional psychiatry and psychoanalysis have devoted their greatest emphasis. We have no good evidence that we can successfully alter the defensive processes of psychotic patients even when great effort is devoted to this task. Perhaps a more indirect and effective route is through building social supports. Here an analogy from the accident field is instructive. Health education programs have thus far found it relatively futile to alter significantly the incidence of automobile accidents through attempts to modify driving behavior. But we know that technological and legal aspects, such as seat belts, highway construction, auto design, and speed limits, have very significant effects on the occurrence of injuries and fatalities (Haddon, Suchman, and Klein, 1964). If there is a technological side to the treatment of the psychoses it lies in how we socially organize the provision and monitoring of drug use and the efforts we make to develop viable networks of services and social support.

4. *Lack of Adequate Social Supports.* It is a truism that men are interdependent, and successful functioning depends on the material assistance and emotional support we receive from our fellows. The absence of such supports makes people vulnerable to interpersonal and environmental assaults and a variety of other adversities (Cobb, 1976; Cassel, 1976). Often the knowledge itself that help is accessible gives people the confidence to cope. But during times of difficulty we depend very heavily on the assistance and moral support of others. Psychotic patients in the community are particularly vulnerable because supports are frequently unavailable. First, such patients often have difficulty in close relationships with others. Second, over the course of time their bizarre behavior and life difficulties have often resulted in the alienation of family and significant others. Third, such patients often fail to maintain contact with services unless the pattern of services is well organized and aggressive. In short,

chronic psychotics are not only very likely to lack such supports, but they also are least likely to effectively seek them out. Although psychoactive drugs are important in the community maintenance of chronic psychotic patients, these patients often fail to maintain their drug therapy and often stop using drugs when their social functioning and psychological state are most tenuous. Without well-organized and aggressive services such patients are often lost in the community and eventually end up in difficulty. Thus far we have had severe problems in developing and maintaining well-organized patterns of supportive care.

5. *Sustained Motivation.* Social adaptation depends on a continuing willingness to remain engaged and on a commitment to ongoing social activities. While withdrawal is a natural and often an effective means of reducing a sense of threat in the short run, it becomes highly maladaptive in a social sense if it persists as a continuing pattern. As people deal with problems by withdrawing, their skills and social contacts tend to erode; and they eventually come to develop a sense of hopelessness.

One of the things we have learned very well in the care of the psychotic patient is that withdrawal and inactivity lead to an erosion of the patient's capacity to continue or to regain important social roles (Wing & Brown, 1970). The specific activity of the patient seems less important than that he remain actively involved, in contact with other people, and constrained to some degree by social expectations. While we have a difficult time unraveling cause from effect, it seems clear that for such patients structure that involves some demands, without overtaxing their ability to conform, contributes to a higher level of social functioning.

In short, I believe that these five areas of inquiry and programming at the level of individual functioning—material resources, skills, defenses, social supports, and sustained motivation—provide a perspective that makes explicit some of the challenges we face. I now turn to a consideration of factors affecting the provision of services and their outcomes.

Social and Social-Psychological Factors Affecting the Provision of Services and their Outcomes

It is well-known that the factors contributing to mental disorders may be different from those leading to social intervention and care or cooperation with treatment programs. The referral of mental patients to services depends on the nature of their manifest symptoms, subcultural tolerance for deviant behavior, and the degree of disturbance caused by the patient in a particular social context (Mechanic, 1968). Similarly, there are wide variations in the extent to which patients or significant others will cooperate with community efforts to assist them. Such problems may be particularly acute in the case of chronic alcoholism, drug addiction, and schizophrenia.

While it is important to understand the social and cultural characteristics that lead patients and their families to resist definitions of disorder and treatment efforts, it is even more crucial for psychiatric services to be aware of how their own patterns of organization may hinder accessibility and effective use of assistance. First, it is necessary to establish that the treatment program itself is one that a reasonable man or woman could wish to take advantage of. Unfortunately, much of the care available for patients with mental impairments could not pass this rather simple test, and one of the contributions of community care innovations is that they offered alternatives to the rather dreary care available in most mental hospitals.

At a more conceptual level, we have learned that health delivery systems, even when they involve no financial barriers to care, erect a variety of other social and psychological barriers that keep certain patients out of their systems or induce a lack of continued participation and cooperation. There is a wide variety of ways in which services come to be rationed: by the resources provided to deal with a given patient load, and the limitations of these resources; by the location of sites of care, and the difficulties involved for patients and their families in reaching such locations; by creating social distance between providers and patients by overprofessionalization and other barriers to communication; by waiting time to obtain services and other noneconomic costs that divert those who particularly have ambivalence about using services to begin with; and by the stigmatization of patients and their families (Mechanic, 1976).

The organization of effective community care in contrast to hospital programs requires a major shift from more traditional bureaucratic perspectives to more organic organizational concepts. While even the most traditional and hierarchical mental hospital organization had to be attuned to some extent to its larger social and political environment, its programs were relatively insulated and separated from community visibility and pressures; and such organizations maintained their own bureaucratic cultures. Although there has been in recent years considerable innovation in staff roles in many of these institutions, the fact is that such hospitals continued to retain relatively rigid professional role structures, and each of the relevant professional groups staked out its own territory and professional routine. The rather marked shift to treatment of psychiatric patients in community voluntary hospitals also followed this bureaucratic emphasis. Indeed, these hospitals are so wedded to the traditional medical model that the psychiatric units tend in their organization to resemble the typical medical services in which different psychiatrists, responsible for varying patients, pass through during the day to make rounds but take little responsibility for the milieu or for dealing with patients' secondary disabilities.

In contrast, effective community care must be exceedingly sensitive to its environment and give attention to such varied concerns as community acceptance, the employment market, the integrity of the welfare and social services system, housing availability, and relationships with police and other social agencies (Mechanic, 1973). Professionals involved in the administration of such programs must be on the scene, their ears to the ground, away from the usual insulation, security, and lack of realism of the professional office. Putting it somewhat differently, the professional in the community care context is a facilitator, coordinator, and integrator. He must become tolerant of more fluid roles and relationships, and be able to work on a more equal basis with a wide range of other mental health professionals as well as with community participants. In this context he is no longer afforded the protection of his medical status or his medical mystique.

Speaking in the lingo of the organizational theorist, there is a variety of reasons explaining why classical models of organizational functioning cannot fit the provision of human services at the community level: the goals are too many and varied and often intangible; the technologies available are not clearly specified and often uncertain; the environment in which programs must operate is unpredictable and changing; the requirements for action in any particular case cannot be unconditionally specified; and the professionals themselves tend to be cosmopolitans with value systems that lead them to reject, subvert, and manipulate traditional bureaucratic rules and structures. In contrast, an organic model of organizational functioning is more attuned to the realities of community care. The name of the game is coordination, and individuals must engage in definition and redefinition of tasks as they relate to others also involved in programming. Responsibilities are fluid and somewhat open-ended, and the task above all requires commitment that goes beyond the application of any particular technical function. Professionals in this context become brokers who must negotiate among varying interests and agencies, and effectiveness resides in the ability to get things done, and not in a traditional authority structure, special degrees, or the mask of medical competence.

In my judgment, the most difficult tasks in any community treatment program are instilling and maintaining a sense of commitment and momentum among program personnel. Community care experiments reported in this volume, although exciting on their own terms, have yet to demonstrate that these programs can maintain their early momentum over long periods of time or communicate their enthusiasm to others. Yet the conditions they treat are chronic and difficult, and often intractable, and require effective and aggressive services over the long range. In the early stages of any new program there is a sense of excitement and innovation. Both personnel and patients feel that something new is being attempted and accomplished. The energy that comes from such involvement is a very powerful treatment force, but it is difficult to maintain over the long haul. People get tired; they seek to regularize their work patterns; they desire to control the uncertainties and unpredictabilities in their environment. Thus they tend to push toward the bureaucratization of roles and the clear-cut definition of responsibilities and turfs; and they become smug about their own failures, less sensitive to the problems of their clients, and less committed to the jobs that have to be done.

I am not aware of any organizational system that has been able to deal effectively with the problem. There are some techniques that are available for encouraging commitment—some less disruptive than others. Perhaps the most typical way in our own society is by recruitment and turnover of personnel. This brings to the organization people who are fresh, enthusiastic, and who have new concepts. In the health services area, however, continuity is essential, and the costs of professional turnover beyond some point may well exceed the benefits. The most viable alternative, in my view, is to maintain a sense of participatory democracy among program personnel. Personnel must be allowed to modify programs from time to time, not so much because the changes themselves will be an improvement, but because participants will feel more enthusiastic about and more committed to programs that they helped formulate and in which they have a stake.

If we have learned nothing else in recent years, we have learned that community care for chronic mental patients, without sustained efforts of follow-up and support, is an invitation to a new type of erosion of human potential, except now it occurs in a community and not in a custodial institution. With the shift to community care we have also learned to what extent professionals can do a disservice to patients under the guise of treatment when they engage in excessive restrictions and foster dependency. We must remain vigilant to the fact that care that encourages dependency rather than incentives to cope can be exceedingly detrimental. Similarly, focusing on life difficulties and symptoms in contrast to potential assets and strengths may reinforce an illness behavior pattern which reduces coping effectiveness. Mental health professionals must never forget that chronicity of illness is one of the few widely and recognized reasons for failing to meet social responsibilities. While mental patients obviously have major handicaps that require persistent and sympathetic professional efforts, the mental health professional must be alert to the possibility that he may be reinforcing ineffective behavior.

The language of social behavior, of course, has moral as well as scientific import. Our language implies a vocabulary of motives, and how we characterize the problems of patients has an impact on their future motives and efforts. One of the major advances of community care has been an increasing tendency to move away from deterministic models of social functioning and to encourage patients to utilize their potential capacities. We must continue to move in this direction but with empathy and avoidance of a crass and cynical behaviorism. The effectiveness of community care will depend on how well we can avoid iatrogenic disabilities without abandoning a humanitarian perspective. The ability to do this depends in large part on forces beyond the control of mental health professionals. It depends on the social and political context of community care, an issue to which I now turn.

The Social and Political Context of Community Care

One of the major difficulties in organizing community environments for the care of the mentally ill is the lack of predictability of the social and political climate. Part of the problem also resides in the fact that we have not yet learned how to successfully balance, or even measure, the social costs for the community against the advantages and ideologies of community care. Despite much rhetoric there is continuing difficulty in maintaining a supportive network of mental health services: in part because of funding problems and the lack of stability in funding patterns; in part because of the difficulty in continuing a sense of innovation and momentum in the care of chronic patients, which is a frustrating task (and a problem I have already discussed); in part because of the difficulties of the reactions and pressures of communities that accept the idea of community care, but in other people's communities; and in part because we often just do not know what we are doing or how to do it.

Anyone involved in serious programming has to be sensitive to the tremendous gap between the enunciation of goals and their implementation. It is one thing to assert a right to treatment; it is quite another to get legislatures to appropriate the funds or to build the network of services required to implement the right. We can talk about less restrictive alternatives and spin legal theories, but it's to no avail if we lack choices in levels or patterns of care. We can theorize about the constructive role of appropriate work in the rehabilitation of mental patients, and its contribution to the sense of dignity and self-esteem of the patient, but we have an uphill battle when ten percent of the labor force is unemployed, and employers face a buyer's market.

As we have moved a larger proportion of patients into community care contexts, we have come face to face with massive resistance of politicians, communities, and neighborhoods. A recent inquiry in California, examining the social functioning of patients in board and care facilities throughout the state, found that the best predictor of their levels of integration was the degree of community acceptance of the facility (Segal and Aviram, 1977). Mental health officials, instead of making efforts to develop an appropriate community climate, often follow the line of least resistance, locating patients in areas that already suffer from disorganization and anomie. Moreover, there is ample indication that a growing number of patients, previously managed within the mental health system, are being processed through the criminal justice system, being charged with minor and vague violations to justify their removal from the community.

If we have learned anything from the history of attempts to desegregate schools and busing, we have learned how difficult it is to translate what we believe to be just and reasonable into workable plans. Certainly, mental health officials must give attention to the concentration of mental patients being relocated in the community, if for no other reason than obvious political desire to avoid a community backlash. While the courts have not sustained the right of a community to pass ordinances to restrict the residence of mental patients, it is hard to believe that a community that wishes to do so can be a very healthy place to carry out programs of community integration. Even the most cursory review of the history of mental health law, I believe, would support the proposition that no matter how wise the courts or how passionate the beliefs of public interest lawyers who have come to the defense of the mentally ill, the development of effective and just solutions depends on the larger context of care and the quality of program alternatives that exist. No legal theory or social ideology, no matter how forceful, can substitute for the willingness of the community to provide the resources for adequate care or for the availability of knowledgeable and committed personnel who are willing to struggle with the frustrating problems involved in providing continuing care on a long-term basis for chronic patients.

We have learned a good deal in the past two decades about the community management of chronic mental disorders. We have learned that, whatever the biological or genetic characteristics of these conditions may be, they can be exacerbated or contained by the manner in which the patients are defined and managed and by the social climate of treatment. We have learned to locate many of the sources of "institutionalism" and factors promoting secondary disabilities. We are making progress in moving from the prevalent concept that a standard therapy fits all mental illness to more careful description and more targeted interventions. We have become more sophisticated about the character of mental disorders and more aware of the labeling process while at the same time avoiding both a glib disease perspective and a crude labeling approach. Perhaps most important of all we have learned how much there is yet to know, and how difficult it is to implement the things we do know. These understandings are the basis of more serious and effective programs of community care in the future.

References

Brenner, H. H. *Mental illness and the economy*. Cambridge: Harvard University Press, 1973.

Cassel, J. The contribution of the social environment to host resistance. *American Journal of Epidemiology*, 104:107–123, 1976.

Cobb, S. Social support as a moderator of life stress. *Psychosomatic Medicine*, 38:300–314, Sept.–Oct., 1976.

Dubos, R. *Mirage of health*. New York: Harper, 1959.

Golann, S., and Fremouw, W. J. (Eds.). *The right to treatment for mental patients*. New York: Irvington, 1976.

Haddon, W. Jr., Suchman, E. A., and Klein, D. (Eds.). *Accident research: methods and approaches*. New York: Harper and Row, 1964.

Mechanic, D. *Medical sociology: a selective view*. New York: The Free Press, 1968.

Mechanic, D. *Mental health and social policy*. Englewood Cliffs, N.J.: Prentice-Hall, 1969.

Mechanic, D. The sociology of organizations, in Saul Feldman (Ed.), *The Administration of Mental Health Services*. Springfield, Ill.: Charles C. Thomas, 1973.

Mechanic, D. *The growth of bureaucratic medicine*. New York: Wiley-Interscience, 1976.

Miller, K. S. *Managing madness: the case against civil commitment*. New York: Free Press, 1976.

Segal, S. P., and Aviram, U. *The mentally ill in community-based sheltered care: a study of community care and social integration*. New York: Wiley-Interscience, 1977.

Wing, J. K., and Brown, G. W. *Institutionalism and schizophrenia*. Cambridge: Cambridge University Press, 1970.

14

Improving the Care of Patients with Chronic Mental Illness

David Mechanic with Linda H. Aiken

The organization of community care for patients with the most severe chronic mental illnesses is seriously deficient. Most of these patients depend exclusively on underfinanced, fragmented, and often inaccessible public services. The difficulties of providing adequate medical and psychiatric services are compounded by homelessness, abuse of alcohol and drugs, and large gaps in the continuum of services necessary to meet the profound needs of these people. Patients lost to the system are commonly found in shelters or jails or on the streets.

Before 1955, when deinstitutionalization began, serious chronic mental illness was treated in public mental hospitals that had responsibility for, and control over, numerous aspects of patients' lives, including their shelter, nutrition, medical care, medication, and daily activities. Many public hospitals, which were substantially overcrowded and understaffed, developed a harsh custodialism that led to vigorous criticism and a devaluation of care in public mental hospitals. Critiques of those hospitals failed to differentiate between poor and good hospital care, and confused common abuses with the important functions of appropriate hospital care.[1]

A variety of technological, cultural, legal, and financial influences reduced patient populations in public mental hospitals from 560,000 patients in 1955 to about 116,000 today. The introduction of neuroleptic drugs in large public hospitals in the middle 1950s controlled the most bizarre manifestations of psychotic illness, gave hospital staff and families hope and a greater sense of control, and increased administrative flexibility. The civil-rights and civil liberties concerns of the 1960s contributed to activism

214

and litigation that extended the rights of the mentally ill and constrained civil commitment. The abuses of the mental hospitals and the criticism of those abuses gave impetus to community care, which was furthered by ideologies of equality, personal autonomy, and environmental determinism. The growth of public welfare programs in the 1960s and the opportunities they provided for states facing economic constraints to shift costs to federal budgets promoted deinstitutionalization. Between 1955 and 1965, the reduction of populations in public hospitals proceeded at a rate of about 1.5 percent per year; between 1965 and 1980, the rate accelerated to approximately 6 percent a year.[2]

Loss of control over the life circumstances of patients diminishes care. Deficiencies in housing, income, basic medical care, and community participation are common and serious. Estimates of the amount of homelessness may vary as much as 10-fold, but studies agree that substantial numbers of homeless persons are psychiatrically impaired and constitute as much as one fourth to two fifths of the homeless population.[3,4] Many patients with chronic illness are impoverished and disoriented and lack basic coping skills, and they require assistance in obtaining disability benefits, Medicaid, and housing. Monitoring drug therapy to maintain necessary medication regimens and to limit severe adverse effects requires care sufficiently aggressive to achieve compliance and to prevent withdrawal and isolation within the community. The care of patients with chronic mental illness is substantially a task of maintenance and rehabilitation that requires longitudinal responsibility and the ability to maintain continuity of care.[5]

The task for effective public mental health systems is one of recreating the functions and responsibilities of the mental hospital in a community context, and this requires highly coordinated services of considerable complexity. Most community systems fail even to approximate this task. It may seem curious that we persist in seeking better organized systems of community care despite many obstacles when we have the alternative of creating good mental hospitals. The community alternative, however, is more consistent with our views of the preciousness of individual autonomy, our beliefs about providing care in the least restrictive setting, and the wishes of patients who prefer deprivations in the community to the restrictions of hospitalization. Moreover, there is much evidence that despite the difficulties, care and rehabilitation services suitable for most patients can be provided in the community and can achieve results superior to those attained in most mental hospitals.[6] Whether this can be done less expensively in the community is more debatable, but comparable funding buys more in the community context.[7]

Effective community care involves the ability to respond to needs

ranging from appropriate housing to medical management of serious psychiatric illness (frequently compounded by other medical problems) requiring a wide range of medical and social services.[8] But psychiatric and
medical leadership in community services for patients with chronic illnesses has seriously declined.[9] Initially, it was believed that community
mental health centers (CMHCs), each of which was responsible for a
particular catchment area, would provide after-care services for patients
discharged from hospitals or serve in lieu of hospitals in the care of
patients with acute psychotic episodes. In their early years, CMHCs failed
to respond to these needs and served large numbers of new clients with
less severe psychiatric problems. At first, there was considerable psychiatric leadership and involvement in CMHCs, but ironically, as these
centers began to direct more of their efforts to the most impaired patients,
medical involvement and responsibility eroded.

The CMHCs, particularly those serving patients receiving public assistance, face many difficulties. With the termination of direct federal funding, they now look to state and local government and third-party payers in
order to survive, and these agencies push the CMHCs in conflicting
directions. By assuming care for the most severely ill patients receiving
public assistance, CMHCs create barriers in regard to the fee-for-service
patients they would like to treat. Because they have limited funds, CMHCs
depend predominantly on psychologists, social workers, nurses, and paraprofessional personnel, who can be recruited at relatively low salaries,
limiting the role of psychiatrists to evaluation and supervision of medication use. Psychiatrists working in these centers have become increasingly
isolated from responsibility for the patients' total care. When given competing and more remunerative opportunities, many have abandoned
CMHCs that serve patients receiving public assistance. Many of the
necessary services for the chronically mentally ill are psychosocial and
are properly carried out by professionals other than psychiatrists, but
there is no justification for the erosion of medical evaluation and supervision as a central component of care.

Case management is vaguely perceived as a solution to many of the
tough issues that plague community care for patients with serious mental
illnesses. This concept has a long tradition in social work, in which case
workers identify and mobilize necessary services on behalf of clients and
may use varying approaches, including street teams, crisis intervention,
and brokering of services. One need only recall the intensive discussion in
medicine of the role of primary care to appreciate the complexity of the
tasks expected of case managers. Typically, case managers assigned to
patients with severe mental illnesses are the lowest-ranking service personnel; they have limited training and experience and little control over the

medical and community resources needed by patients. The pay is low, career ladders are nonexistent, and attrition is high. It is foolish to place so much hope on an intervention that is as weak as this one and has so little supporting structure. If case management is to be effective, it must be embedded in an organizational strategy that clearly defines who is responsible for care, that has in place the necessary service elements to provide the full spectrum of needed services, and that can control a range of resources so that balanced decisions can be made. The remainder of this discussion will address these strategies.

Community tolerance of the mentally ill has diminished in the absence of decent services. The public mental health sector must be revitalized if we are to avoid the recreation of public asylums. Building an effective public system will take dedicated professional commitment, a focused planning and organizational structure, and a new way of consolidating public financing. There is a compelling need for psychiatrists to become involved in the public sector and to provide the essential medical management.

Unlike public mental hospitals, or typical medical outpatient systems, public mental health services must reach patients in a variety of settings, including shelters, the streets, board and care facilities, and jails. Services have to be more aggressive than those typically provided and less dependent on the initiative and appreciation of those served. The service system, whether through direct services, contracts, or coordinating mechanisms, should have the capacity to negotiate needs for housing, social welfare benefits, medical evaluation, medication maintenance, rehabilitation services, and the like. In most urban areas, however, the responsibility for such services is divided among various levels of government, and service agencies are financed by diverse sources.

A key element in any effort to improve community services is to capture more hospital funds for programs of managed care at the local level that are responsible for both inpatient and outpatient services for defined populations. Some regions are establishing mental health boards, nonprofit mental health corporations, public authorities, and other types of legal entities that are responsible for receiving and disbursing mental health funds from diverse sources, including state and local governments, Medicaid, and private insurance (Walsh AH, Leigland J: unpublished data). Wisconsin, for example, provides state funding to local county mental health boards, which either directly provide or purchase all outpatient and inpatient care for mentally ill residents.[10] Savings achieved by preventing unnecessary hospitalization are available to finance innovative community care models for persons with severe mental illnesses. Ohio has developed a legal framework for strong local mental health boards and is considering legislation to divert funding traditionally allocated to state mental hospitals to these boards for more comprehensive management of care. Several areas, including Philadelphia, Rochester, New York, and South Carolina, are in varying stages of implementing limited capitation approaches for the chronically mentally ill. With the assistance of $100 million in resources from the Robert Wood Johnson Foundation and the U.S. Department of Housing and Urban Development, nine large cities are developing mental health authorities intended to have the capacity to cope with financial and organizational fragmentation.[11]

Consolidating resources across inpatient and outpatient services is particularly difficult in states with entrenched hospital systems, in communities that are economically dependent on such hospitals, and in areas with well-organized and unionized hospital employees. The need to maintain the stability of existing hospital services and to achieve necessary political support argues for transition strategies aimed at shifting funding directions over a certain period. A well-organized system diverts inappropriate admissions to suitable community programs and makes provisions for discharge planning soon after hospital admission.

Except for state mental health budgets (67 percent of which are used to maintain hospitals[12]), Medicaid constitutes the largest potential funding source for reorganizing the financing of care for the severely mentally ill population. Federal Medicaid contributions represent more than two thirds of all federal funds received by state mental health agencies,[12] and in 1983, Medicaid contributed $991 million for care in state and county mental hospitals.[13] In addition, most Medicaid funds for mental health services are spent outside the control of public mental health administrators or a managed system of mental health care. In 1980, Medicaid was the expected principal source of payment for 23 percent of all psychiatric admissions to nonfederal general hospitals and for 7 percent of all admissions to private psychiatric hospitals.[12] A rough estimate suggests that in 1980 Medicaid was the expected principal source of payment for 1.9 million bed-days in nonfederal general hospitals and private psychiatric institutions and that approximately two thirds of these bed-days were for patients with chronic mental illnesses. Patients with such illnesses come or are brought by police to emergency rooms, where they are seen by physicians who are unfamiliar with them and who, because of the insecurities that uncertainty provokes, choose hospitalization, which is often financed by Medicaid. In a well-organized system, many of these admissions could be prevented and the patient referred to more appropriate community services.

Reforming Medicaid in this context would be complex, but managed care for Medicaid patients with chronic mental illnesses that is also supported by capitated state mental health funding holds considerable promise. Surles and McGurrin[14] found that in Philadelphia, persons who frequently use facilities providing emergency psychiatric services typically use the facilities as a point of entry to the mental health system. Moreover, although such patients account for only 20 percent of the unduplicated caseload, they use 60 percent of all service hours and constitute 55 percent of all admissions. These patients are not part of an organized program appropriate for their needs, and their unpredictable episodic use of services causes crises in the system and is extremely costly. Officials in Philadelphia are making efforts to negotiate a capitation program with state and federal Medicaid authorities to manage the care of such high-risk patients in order to provide appropriate psychiatric care in conjunction with sophisticated psychosocial services. They believe they can do so within the current range of expenditures for these patients.

There are many uncertainties in capitation, but careful demonstrations that allow better management of expenditures for defined populations of patients at high risk must go forward. In 1986, Congress made specific provisions for such managed-care waivers in Medicaid-financed mental health services. Unlike the situation in traditional managed-care systems (health maintenance organizations [HMOs]), which share risks among enrollees, the objective of the new systems is to provide meaningful trade-offs among types of care for a population of high-risk patients. Thus, the design of a managed-care system for these patients should not be confused with the inclusion of patients with chronic mental illnesses into mainstream HMOs, where such patients typically do not fare well.[15] The idea of capitated care targeted to patients with chronic mental illnesses requires a sophisticated and responsible mental health entity that has the authority and organizational capacity to balance community and inpatient care, as well as psychiatric and social services. In many communities, the framework and spectrum of necessary services are deficient, but managed care contributes to a resource base and incentive to develop the necessary components of service into a system.

Building a strong organizational structure that can give coherence to the system of services for the chronically mentally ill is central to the types of tasks that must be addressed if a true alternative for hospitalization is to be developed on a broad basis. The effectiveness of doing so has been demonstrated in selected programs and in some controlled clinical trials.[6, 16–18] The Stein and Test "training in community living" model, which combines aggressive psychiatric community care with case management and training in psychosocial skills, has been partly or entirely adopted in a number of communities.[19] In the period 1979 to 1981, the model was replicated in Sydney, Australia, and evaluated in a randomized controlled trial. The outcomes were favorable as compared with those achieved with traditional care.[20] At the 12-month follow-up, for example, almost two thirds of the patients who had received the experimental treatment were very satisfied, as compared with less than one third of controls. Similarly, 83 percent of the relatives of patients in the experimental-treatment group with whom the patients lived were very satisfied with treatment, as compared with 26 percent of the controls.

The challenge is to learn how to adapt successful models developed in smaller communities to more complex urban, political, and professional environments. The Sydney experience suggests that such an effort is feasible. In a recent review, Kiesler and Sibulkin[21] identified 14 experimental studies, most of which incorporated random assignment, demonstrating that community alternatives were more effective than hospitalization across a wide range of patient populations and treatment strategies. Substantial organizational barriers persist. The catchment-area concept that has dominated community mental health services divides large cities into multiple relatively autonomous services units. Within a catchment-area framework, chronically ill patients are easily lost to follow-up, and the limited population base makes it difficult to organize specialized services, such as jail diversion and programs for patients with multiple illnesses and for homeless mentally ill persons. In addition, the mental health system typically is not in a position in the structure of local governments to allow it to influence non-health-related local services required to build an effective alternative to hospital care. Often, mental health services remain under the jurisdiction of the state government, whereas public housing, welfare, and police services necessary for effective psychiatric emergency response systems are controlled by the city or county government. The challenge is to integrate services at the local level without diminishing existing state financial obligations.

Since housing is a particularly critical element in developing an alternative to hospital care, it serves as an example of the gap between the present and potential opportunities. Mental health agencies in large cities have limited available housing placements, despite the facts that homelessness is an acute problem among mentally ill persons and that housing is an integral part of the therapeutic care plan. In many of our largest cities, as little as 5 to 10 percent of the estimated housing placements needed are available to the mental health services system. A range of housing options, from supervised group homes and apartments to scattered site locations, is essential. Many chronically mentally ill persons are eligible for housing assistance but receive little attention from city housing authorities who have no understanding of their special needs, or from mental health centers who have limited understanding of how to garner a larger share of public housing resources. A strong local mental health entity could develop sufficient expertise in housing to collaborate more effectively with the public housing authority and nonprofit developers in order to initiate joint ventures to provide suitable housing opportunities for this population. The availability of crisis support for landlords has been useful in achieving successful housing placements in the Training for Community Living Program in Dane County, Wisconsin,[19] and in community programs in Boston managed by the Massachusetts Mental Health Center.[22] In reality, this is not a large service burden, but the promise that help, if needed, is available on a 24-hour basis gives landlords, employers, police, and others sufficient confidence to cooperate. Such efforts have not been attempted in many larger cities, and the approach still requires evaluation.

The success of programs in each of the above areas has been demonstrated in one setting or another, but rarely do such programs come together in a single community. The difficulty of consolidating the necessary administrative authority, control over financing, and complex intraorganizational relations necessary is an important part of our present crisis and future challenge. An effectively constituted public organization with the ability to direct substantial resources and with credibility would make it possible to link components essential for maintenance of function and rehabilitation into a responsible and effective alternative to care in a mental hospital.

References

1. Mechanic D. Mental health and social policy. 2nd ed. Englewood Cliffs, N.J.: Prentice-Hall, 1980.
2. Gronfein W. Incentives and intentions in mental health policy: a comparison of the Medicaid and Community Mental Health programs. J. Health Soc Behav 1985; 26:192–206.
3. Lamb HR, ed. The homeless mentally ill: a task force report of the American Psychiatric Association. Washington, D.C.: American Psychiatric Association, 1984.
4. Rossi PH, Wright JD, Fisher GA, Willis G. The urban homeless: estimating composition and size. Science 1987; 235:1336–41.
5. Mechanic D. The challenge of chronic mental illness: a retrospective and prospective view. Hosp Community Psychiatry 1986; 37:891–6.
6. Stein LI, Test MA, eds. Alternatives to mental hospital treatment. New York: Plenum Press, 1978.
7. Weisbrod BA, Test MA, Stein LI. Alternatives to mental hospital treatment. II. Economic benefit-cost analysis. Arch Gen Psychiatry 1980; 37:400–5.
8. Mechanic D. Correcting misconceptions in mental health policy: strategies for improved care of the seriously mentally ill. Milbank Q 1987; 65:203–30.
9. Faulkner LR, Bloom JD, Bray JD, Maricle R. Medical services in community mental health programs. Hosp Community Psychiatry 1986; 37:1045–7.
10. Stein LI, Ganser LJ. Wisconsin system for funding mental health services. In:

Talbott J, ed. New directions for mental health services: unified mental health systems. San Francisco: Jossey-Bass, 1983:25–32.

11. Aiken LH, Somers SA, Shore MF. Private foundations in health affairs: a case study of the development of a national initiative for the chronically mentally ill. Am Psychol 1986; 41:1290–5.

12. Taube CA, Barrett SA, eds. Mental health, United States, 1985. Washington, D.C.: Government Printing Office, 1985. (DHHS publication no. (ADM) 85–1378.)

13. Redick RW, Witkin MJ, Atay JE, Manderscheid BW. Specialty mental health organizations, United States, 1983–84. Washington, D.C.: Government Printing Office, 1986. (DHHS publication no. (ADM) 86–1490.)

14. Surles RC, McGurrin MC. Increased use of psychiatric emergency services by young chronic mentally ill patients. Hosp Community Psychiatry 1987; 38:401–5.

15. Schlesinger M. On the limits of expanding health care reform: chronic care in prepaid settings. Milbank Q 1986; 64:189–215.

16. Falloon IRH, Boyd JL, McGill CW, et al. Family management in the prevention of morbidity of schizophrenia: clinical outcomes of a two-year study. Arch Gen Psychiatry 1985; 42:887–96.

17. Stein LI, Test MA. Alternatives to mental hospital treatment. I. Conceptual model, treatment program, and clinical evaluation. Arch Gen Psychiatry 1980; 37:392–7.

18. Leff J, Kuipers L, Berkowitz R, Eberlein-Vries R, Sturgeon D. A controlled trial of social intervention in the families of schizophrenic patients. Br J Psychiatr 1982; 141:121–34.

19. Stein LI, Test MA, eds. Training in community living model: a decade of experience. New directions for mental health services, no. 26. San Francisco: Jossey-Bass, 1985.

20. New South Wales, Department of Health. Psychiatric hospital versus community treatment: a controlled study. Sydney, Australia: Department of Health, 1983. (HSR 83–046.)

21. Kiesler CA, Sibulkin AE. Mental hospitalization: myths and facts about a national crisis. Newbury Park, Calif.: Sage, 1987.

22. Gudeman JE, Shore MF. Beyond deinstitutionalization: a new class of facilities for the mentally ill. N Engl J Med 1984; 311:832–6.

15

Challenges in Long-Term Care Policy

The health care arena is in extraordinary ferment.[1] The traditional structures that have defined medical practice, such as the hospital and solo physician practice, are undergoing major transformations, but the shape of future organization is still in an early stage of evolution. The realignments now taking place are experienced as major dislocations by providers and managers of existing services, but there is little reason to anticipate that adequately insured consumers will experience dramatic differences in patterns of care or in the responsiveness of health services. The biggest challenges for the system will be maintaining services for the uninsured and for patients covered by public programs facing fiscal pressures and responding to the emerging needs of an increasingly elderly population.

The obvious strains are most likely to be felt in the public sector, and particularly in the financing and administration of the Medicare and Medicaid programs. Also, as more of the population enters the ages associated with disability and dependence, our failure to develop a coherent policy of long-term care that protects the elderly and their families at the period of greatest vulnerability will increase in salience and will become a more explosive social issue. We would do well to face the restructuring of Medicare and Medicaid, and the development of long-term care policies now, before the demographic and financial implications push us into expedient but poorly conceived solutions.

The Demographic Scenario

The awesome scenario of the aging of the American population, and its implications for dependency and medical and social services costs, are now commonplace. The population aged sixty-five years and over has increased from 8.1 percent in 1950 to approximately 12 percent now, and will continue to increase moderately until 2010, when this age group will constitute almost 14 percent of the population. In the subsequent two decades as the postwar birth cohorts reach age sixty-five, the proportion is expected to increase to approximately 21 percent. The population age seventy-five and older, now constituting two-fifths of those over sixty-five, will increase to almost half in the next twenty-five years.[2]

Age distribution is largely a product of the size of varying age cohorts and changing patterns of mortality. Trends in these demographic patterns result in dramatic increases in the numbers of elderly eighty-five years or older. Between 1960 and 1980 this subgroup increased faster than any other age group, and is expected to constitute almost 15 percent of those over sixty-five within the next fifteen years.[3] The proportion of persons reaching age sixty-five who attain age eighty-five increased from 23 percent in 1950 to 38 percent in 1983.[4]

Projections into the future, based on present patterns, are always a hazardous endeavor. We have been less than accurate in anticipating changes in social and political values, new knowledge and technologies, trends in economic well-being, attitudes toward income redistribution, and the occurrence of new epidemics. As we project into the future, we can be confident that our extrapolations from the past will be faulty, but failure to plan seriously for the inevitable would be foolish indeed.

Barring extraordinary and unexpected events, the changing age distribution, and particularly the growing numbers at ages where chronic illness and limitation of function are common, will put significant pressures on our systems of social welfare and entitlements. It may be that changing risks throughout the lifespan will lead to some compression of morbidity— a debatable hypothesis.[5] However, even if the period of chronic illness and incapacity is compressed, the magnitude of the overall burden of illness will be well beyond our experience. Demographic patterns, together with scientific and technological capabilities to sustain life, already strain our social welfare structures, but we still have the luxury of some time to plan intelligently for the momentous challenges as the baby boom generations move into their later years.

With an aging society, attention is focused commonly on rates of dependency in the population and ratios of those of typical employment age relative to others. Inevitably, this suggests alarm about the falling proportion of workers relative to the population. Such ratios, projected over time, are not particularly meaningful without careful consideration of the likely trends in automation in the production of goods and services, advances in computer technologies and robotics, the number of children, and possible changes in norms and values about who should work. Growth of female participation in the labor force made projections based on earlier norms meaningless, and we need not assume that either retirement age or its downward trend is immutable. While retirements prior to age sixty-five are increasing, the factors motivating such behavior could change substantially with altered views of the lifespan, economic pressures and incentives, and new conceptions of what it means to be elderly.

It is surprisingly, for example, that so little attention has been given to how immigration policy over the next fifty years might help insulate the society from shocks associated with a less than optimal age distribution. Immigration policy has set quotas in relation to varying nations, occupational strata, and relationships to U.S. citizens. In theory, an immigration policy planned over a couple of decades could help smooth the age distribution to moderate some of the most alarming consequences of an aging society. This would substantially deviate from current policy and trends, but the use of immigration policy as an instrument for demographic balance is one of many possible strategies for an aging society.

The Implications of Aging for Health Care Planning

The health status of varying birth cohorts as they approach the later years reflects a broad history of personal habits and environmental influences throughout the lifespan. There is indication that successive cohorts at different ages in middle and later life are more healthy, possibly a product of improved living conditions during their development or a result of positive health behavior that reduces exposure to risk factors. Aggregate data on health status and illness by age are not particularly informative because the inclusion of persons whose mortality is reduced or delayed through sophisticated medical measures inflates aggregate overall rates of illness and disability, which may mask other improvements in health status in the population.[6] Increased longevity of elderly populations with serious chronic illness, however, poses serious challenges for the provision of medical and other long-term care services. As individuals move into the eighth and ninth decades of life, the probability of decreased function, dependence on others, and risk of institutionalization substantially increases. Thus, the number of individuals at risk, while only a small portion of those over sixty-five, is a relatively large segment at age eighty-five.[7]

Long-term care for the elderly is substantially rationed by the abhorrence many elderly have for residence in nursing homes. Persons who could meet any reasonable criteria for nursing home admission hang on with the assistance of family, friends, and neighbors to avoid entering institutions. The trigger for admission is often not the level of need alone, a criterion that could be met by many living outside nursing homes, but rather the loss of a spouse or other significant supportive persons or a major illness or accident that makes persons lacking supports unable to care for themselves.

There is a perversity about a system of care that depends for its equilibrium on public abhorrence. Those elderly with significant needs for care greatly outnumber those in nursing homes. For many such patients, home and community care are preferable, and in the individual instance, economical as well. But shifting services to the community removes the barrier of abhorrence, opening increased demand that promises aggregate long-term care costs in excess of current expenditures. Herein lies the dilemma and the challenge that a prudent and humane public policy must address.

Policy Issues at the Federal Level

Cost-containment pressures affect government programs acutely be-cause the federal government pays a large proportion of total health expenditures (28.9 percent in 1983), because health care costs constitute a significant component of the federal budget (over 12 percent in 1983), and because health expenditures make up even a larger proportion of the federal budget under administrative and legislative control. Given its magnitude and discretionary possibilities, it becomes an area of close scrutiny in times of budgetary constraint. Projections of the expected insolvency of the Medicare Trust Fund have been pushed forward as the economy has improved, but demographic realities will require us to reassess the future structure of Medicare, and to face the inadequacies of long-term care provision.

Ideally, we seek a program that eases access to high-quality care among those who most need care; distributes entitlements in an equitable way; protects vulnerable individuals and their families against catastrophic costs; and shapes incentives for professionals, patients, and caretakers to promote improved function and rehabilitation efforts. Notwithstanding the ambiguity of such terms as access, quality, need, and equity, it seems clear that in addition to Parts A and B (hospital costs and physicians' services, respectively), as currently constituted, Medicare should include protection against catastrophic acute care costs. But this is only a small part of the problem. A strategy for long-term care is required that makes it possible for the most needy to obtain care without first impoverishing themselves or their families, a common occurrence in many jurisdictions under Medicaid regulations. Medicare costs cover only 44 percent of health care costs of the elderly, and recipients now contribute a larger proportion of income out-of-pocket than they did prior to 1966 when the program was implemented. In some subgroups, such expenditures exceed acceptable levels of total income.[8]

The Responsibility of the Elderly

As we examine ways of reducing cost sharing for those with least income, there is also merit in examining carefully the capacity of some elderly to take responsibility for greater costs as a way of protecting and enhancing the benefit structure. Alternative approaches include taxing the value of the Medicare benefit among recipients whose incomes exceed a defined ceiling, eliminating other preferences to the high-income elderly, or taxing more Social Security income above a specified income level. Means testing is increasingly suggested but would alter the program irrevocably. The beauty of Medicare is its universality and its acceptance and support across all social groups in the population. Unlike Medicaid, it is not a welfare program and is immune to the stigma and distrust commonly associated with the Title XIX program.

The obvious needs to address catastrophic costs and to plan more appropriately for long-term care would suggest greater dependence on general revenues. In the context of a large deficit, an ideology supporting the contraction of the federal government, and resistance to increased taxes, this is no easy matter, and identifying ways to reduce program expenditures will continue to be the main emphasis of public policy. In the absence of increased revenues, there are four general alternatives: changing eligibility criteria to reduce the pool of beneficiaries, increased cost sharing, continued tightening of reimbursement, and modifying the benefit structure. Most of these alternatives are not desirable, but we probably will see efforts in all of these areas.

The problems of Medicare and Medicaid are not isolated issues but should be seen in the context of health subsidies in general. Recently, Enthoven estimated that the tax subsidy of health insurance benefits was almost $50 billion and likely to increase as a result of a recent Internal Revenue Service (IRS) ruling permitting health insurance premium contributions to be purchased with before-tax dollars when certain conditions are met.[9] While some subsidy encouraging health care insurances is defensible, existing subsidies have encouraged overinsurance among the affluent, which, if we take the Rand Health Insurance results seriously, contributes little to improved health status but increases utilization and cost.[10]

There is broad recognition of the inequity of this subsidy, but those who benefit from it have been effective in resisting its modification. Revision may be more feasible, however, within a framework that reallocates the subsidy to address such issues as catastrophic costs, long-term care, and the needs of the uninsured and those institutions that provide much of their care. Reducing a tax benefit to lower federal expenditures may be less compelling than devising a more equitable and acceptable framework for care overall. The latter, if well designed, could coalesce a range of influential constituencies that could potentially provide the necessary political momentum.

The Role of Public Financing

A major challenge is to maintain the universality of Medicare, but in a context that offers broader protection against catastrophe and a mode of financing that protects low-income recipients from burdensome levels of cost sharing. The increased cost sharing in Medicare involving an inpatient deductible of $520 for each period of illness, a $75 deductible and 20 percent coinsurance for approved doctors' charges, and heavy coinsurance for hospital stays exceeding sixty days has led to devastating costs in individual instances. Approximately two-thirds of Medicare patients protect themselves by purchasing Medigap insurance that covers much of these costs, but such policies are expensive relative to the benefits provided because of marketing, administrative costs, and profits. Medicare could provide expanded benefits at no greater cost than the elderly now pay for Medigap protection. This approach was suggested by the Social Security Advisory Council, and recent legislation has substantially increased catastrophic coverage for medical care but most of long-term care needs are not covered.

The 30 million Medicare recipients are a highly varied group, economically and otherwise. Disparities in income are large and tend to be underestimated, since affluent elderly receive a larger proportion of their resources from unearned income that is not fully reported.[11] A significant proportion of elderly have modest incomes (approximately half within 200 percent of the poverty line) but are not sufficiently destitute to be eligible for Medicaid.[12] Thus, health expenditures may usurp an intolerable proportion of their income, preventing them from fulfilling other needs. One approach to remedying the uneven result of cost sharing is to provide a tax credit to recipients whose out-of-pocket health expenditures exceed some reasonable proportion of income. Those whose incomes, in contrast, exceed specified levels could be taxed on the average value of the Medicare benefit.

Much attention has been focused on efforts to tighten reimbursement under Medicare and the implementation and consequences of Medicare's prospective payment system (PPS). The growth of physician payment under Medicare Part B has also stimulated a variety of measures to control physician payment, including a freeze on fee increases. (Payment to physicians increased 106 percent between 1979–83, almost three times the gross national product.[13]) The unwillingness of many physicians to accept Medicare assignment puts the burden of payment on the elderly for charges beyond those allowable by Medicare. This can substantially inflate required out-of-pocket expenditures. Various proposals are being considered to encourage physicians to accept assignment, as well as mandatory assignment approaches.[14] There is concern that mandatory assignment would make physicians less accessible to the elderly, but, given the important contribution Medicare makes to physician income, the growing numbers of physicians, and the increasing competition for patients, it seems unlikely that many physicians would opt out of Medicare. Measuring the quality and responsiveness of care, in contrast, is more difficult, but fears about diminished attention to patients with mandatory assignment constraints, particularly in light of the increasing competitiveness of the arena, may be exaggerated.

Medicare's PPS constitutes a stage in the evolution of a more comprehensive prospective payment system. On the one hand, more thought is being given to extending the PPS approach to other services, such as nursing home payment and inpatient physician services. On the other hand, serious efforts are being made to enroll the elderly into capitated arrangements, such as health maintenance organizations (HMOs), in which the health entity assumes the risks of unanticipated costs. PPS, as it now operates, is simply a tool to control payments. We can anticipate increased efforts to refine diagnosis-related groups (DRGs) to control for complexity of care. Also, we can expect reduced payments as economic pressures in the program increase and better hospital performance data that justify modifications become available.

Hospital and physician reimbursement policies reflect the need to control program costs and, it is hoped, to encourage efficiency, but processes of decisionmaking within the hospital remain uncertain. It is not obvious that constraints result in wise decisions or that managers in hospitals have the authority to constrain physician behavior constructively. With the increased availability of physicians, managers have more options, yet their dependence on physicians' patients in a highly competitive situation has countervailing influences. We need a much better, more detailed understanding of how decisions are worked out in this context. Peer Review Organizations and other regulatory authorities, and the rapidity of change, add to the reasons to anticipate major gaps between theory about the internal responses of hospitals and reality.

Strategies for Long-Term Care

In the absence of a national strategy for long-term care, and the exclusion of long-term services from Medicare coverage, Medicaid, by default, constitutes our national long-term care program, financing approximately half of national nursing homes expenditures. The cost of long-term care taxes the resources of most families, and typically elderly entrants to nursing homes on their own resources spend down until they reach eligibility for Medicaid. In the case of a family unit, however, the patient's elderly spouse is commonly forced into poverty before eligibility is reached, a situation that shocks the conscience of the public. The problems of building a long-term care constituency are exacerbated by the common belief among the public that Medicare provides needed protection. Four-fifths of members surveyed by the American Association of Retired Persons, who thought they might require long-term care in the future, believed that all or most of the costs were covered by Medicare or private insurance.

Community-Based Care

The goal is to develop an appropriate strategy for financing long-term care within a framework that enhances continued participation and function in the community to the greatest extent possible, and reinforces the informal care and supports that currently exist. When home care is no longer feasible because of mental confusion, incontinence, and extreme disability, and when the burdens on caretakers become too large, we seek a competent and caring institutional environment.

Considerable consensus exists on goals, but the enormous potential costs of long-term care give most policymakers reason to pause. More attention is now being given to the potential of long-term care insurance and community organizational structures that can bring together and coordinate a broader range of care needed by the frail elderly.[15] The current social health maintenance organization (SHMO) demonstrations supported by the Health Care Financing Administration (HCFA) should provide useful information on the viability of this approach.

Intuitively, it seems plausible that if we appropriately organize home and community services for the elderly, we should be able to provide high-quality care at a cost comparable to or less than that of institutional care. But what seems intuitively plausible is not necessarily true, and we have much to learn about how better to target individuals truly at risk of institutionalization who can, with appropriate services, remain in the community.[16] Moreover, when individuals are sufficiently debilitated and confused, and require sophisticated services and high levels of supervision, instituional care may be the less expensive alternative. Similarly, the burden on caretakers must be factored into consideration. In short, we need better concepts of triage that identify what patients and needs are most appropriately cared for in varying service contexts.

Cost per person must be differentiated from aggregate costs for populations. Most elderly hang on in the community as long as possible. But an attractive community/home care benefit brings new clients, who contribute to a higher aggregate cost. Such benefits often become complements rather than substitutes. These new clients who are attracted to community care benefits are in need but less disabled than those at high risk of institutionalization. Patients with such characteristics who enter nursing homes frequently return to their own homes after a relatively short stay.[17] Thus, while community care may be preferable, it must be justified on the basis of community values and quality of care, and not as a cost-saving alternative.

Eligibility Screening

If long-term care needs are to be met by a broader set of options than now exists, and at tolerable cost, then screening for eligibility for services must be an important component of any program. Sophisticated evaluation is essential, but screening costs can be expensive because those at risk are a small proportion of the frail. The preservation of informal supports is extremely important, but can be undermined if programming strategy is not mindful of the extent to which community sustenance depends on this hidden system of care. Incentives can reinforce and strengthen these informal networks by helping reduce burdens on caretakers and providing respite opportunities.

Sources of Funding

If long-term care financing is to be responsive to the evolving need, then various sources of funding will be necessary. Future cohorts of elderly will have more resources in the form of pensions and other assets, and there is growing interest in such mechanisms as long-term care insurance, long-term care individual retirement accounts (IRAs), and reverse mortgages. Structuring a combination of these mechanisms, along with direct governmental support, is a complex endeavor involving a variety of questions for which good data are not easily available. Despite strong constraints on the long-term care sector, it has grown rapidly. Nursing home care increased from less than 2 percent to 9 percent of personal

health care costs, between 1950 and 1983, with estimated expenditures of
$35 billion in 1985.[18] Approximately 46 percent of expenditures come from
public sources, with more than two-thirds from federal programs, primarily
Medicaid. Long-term care services provided in the community and home
are difficult to disaggregate from other health and social services in the
community, but still constitute a small fraction of long-term care expenditures.

The dilemma faced by both public and private programs is how to
expand long-term care services and better respond to community needs
within acceptable economic limits without unleashing a high level of
demand that exceeds the capacity or willingness of the community to pay.
The problem is somewhat different for the affluent with assets, who might
buy long-term care protection through private insurance, life care community residence, or other means, and the majority of elderly with limited
assets who inevitably must depend on public programs. But, in either
case, mechanisms must be in place to assure the viability of economic
arrangements.

Rationing Services

The strategies for rationing long-term care services are comparable to
those used in the health sector generally. But because they involve skills
and services that can be more easily met by informal sources such as
homemaker assistance, chore services, meal preparation, transportation,
and some home nursing services, the potential for shifting informal costs
to programs is large. This presents difficult actuarial problems and encourages restrictive insurance options. Any adequate long-term care provision
probably would require considerable cost sharing not only to reduce the
obligation of third-party payers but also to establish a threshold beyond
which persons who have alternative informal sources are less likely to
seek benefits. Deductibles and coinsurance must not be so large as to
inhibit the provision of essential services, but must be large enough so that
there is no obvious incentive for family and friends to shift responsibility.
This is an exceedingly difficult issue because objectives are in conflict and
defining the proper balance of incentives is fraught with uncertainty.

An alternative or complement is to have case managers make decisions
about benefits through the application of screening criteria. Such judgments about community and home services are far more uncertain than
are decisions about nursing home admission, and much effort is needed in
perfecting such criteria. The task is more difficult than decisions about
necessary medical services, and requires judgments not only about what
persons can do on their own, but also about the strengths and capabilities

of their families and extended informal networks. This task, thus, is inextricably associated with complex personal and social values, norms about the obligations of the family, notions about what friends owe to one another, and the like. The area thus involves difficult ethical issues and assessments and is highly vulnerable to the excesses of discretion and inequitable outcomes. We should learn something about this process from the ongoing. SHMO demonstrations, but the inherent problems are not easily solved. Discretion can be contained to some degree by specifying in detail the conditions under which varying types of services would be available. The exercise might be informative for those managing such a program, but it is difficult to visualize how the complex judgments involved can be prescribed sensibly.

Long-Term Care and Society

Long-term care is a social process, more so than is the provision of traditional health care as we usually view it. It depends to a larger degree on notions of community, networks of reciprocal obligation, and competing and changing values among the generations. In a narrow sense, the challenge of long-term care is in developing a financial structure that assures that the pressing needs of the sick and disabled elderly will be met. But any viable financing structure must be developed within a meaningful community context and consistent with efforts to sustain voluntary efforts.

For those elderly who lose their capacity for social relations as a consequence of Alzheimer's disease, stroke, or other devastating infirmities, the major challenge is financing the care that informal sources are unable to give without insufferable burden. But for many disabled elderly, the challenge is to sustain their function and participation and to maintain their sense of self and personal dignity. Thus, the source of care, and how it is provided, is no small issue. If the elderly view the substitute of formal care for informal services, whatever the quality, as a betrayal by loved ones and the community, the results will be deficient.

While most elderly prefer community to institutional care, their desire to avoid financial dependence on their children is highly prevalent and has increased over time.[19] Thus, it seems plausible that as the population contemplates increased longevity and the prospects of aging, and becomes better educated about the inadequacy of long-term care protections, it will be more prepared to invest in protecting against the risks of incapacity and dependence. Approximately one in five of those over sixty-five now require nursing home care, but as the demographic composition of the elderly group changes, needs for care will increase. If the risk is sufficiently spread over the population, the burden on any individual need not be excessive.

Possibilities for long-term care coverage range from mandatory program participation through an extension of the social security system to private long-term insurance embodied in employee benefit plans or purchased on the open market. To the extent that such coverage is not mandatory, the usual problems of marketing, risk selection, and public education are major concerns, and leave open the question of how we care for those who lack the necessary prudence or who play the odds in addition to those who lack the economic resources to protect themselves.

Ironically, our society has the facilities, the capacity, and the human resources necessary to ensure our population decent care. With our abundant institutional capacity, our growing corps of physicians, nurses, social workers, and other health professionals, and our strong tradition of volunteerism, we have the necessary components for a comprehensive and vital response to the challenges. The growing elderly population itself is a major resource than can contribute immensely with creative organization. Many retired persons seek fruitful opportunities to serve others and to maintain their sense of meaningful participation. We have yet to develop appropriate organizational contexts on a wide scale that can utilize this rich reservoir of productive activity.

Long-term care must be seen not simply as a medical or custodial problem, or solely within the larger context of providing social services. Effective long-term care requires major initiatives in social organization and the modification of community culture along with the health and social services that those with impaired function require. It is through a balance of increased public entitlements, nongovernmental initiatives, enhanced voluntary efforts, and individual responsibility of the elderly and their families that we have an opportunity to provide not only the critical services that a decent society demands, but also a framework that gives the later years meaning and dignity.

Notes

1. D. Mechanic, *From Advocacy to Allocation: The Evolving American Health Care System* (New York: Free Press, 1986).
2. J. S. Siegel and C. M. Taeuber, "Demographic Perspectives on the Long-Lived Society," *Daedalus* 115 (1986):82.
3. Office of Technology Assessment, *Technology and Aging in America*, OTA-BA-264 (Washington, D.C.: U.S. Congress OTA, 1985):42.
4. Siegel and Taeuber, "Demographic Perspectives on the Long-Lived Society," 90.
5. E. Schneider and J. Brody, "Aging, Natural Death, and the Compression of

Morbidity: Another View," *The New England Journal of Medicine* 309 (1984):854–855.

6. L. Verbrugge, "Longer Life But Worsening Health Trends in Health and Mortality of Middle-Aged and Older Persons," *Milbank Memorial Fund Quarterly* 62 (1984):475–519.

7. R. Suzman and M. W. Riley, eds., "Special Issue: The Oldest Old," *Milbank Memorial Fund Quarterly* 63 (1985).

8. K. Davis, "Aging and the Health Care System: Economic and Structural Issues." *Daedalus* 115 (1986):227–246.

9. A. Enthoven, "Health Tax Policy Mismatch," *Health Affairs* (Winter 1985):5–14.

10. R. H. Brook et al., "Does Free Care Improve Adults' Health?: Results from a Randomized Controlled Trial," *The New England Journal of Medicine* 309 (1983):1426–1434.

11. S. Crystal, "Measuring Income and Inequality Among the Elderly," *The Gerontologist* 26 (1986):56–59.

12. Davis, "Aging and the Health Care System," 231.

13. R. H. Arnett III et al., "Health Spending Trends in the 1980s: Adjusting to Financial Incentives," *Health Care Financing Review* 6 (1985):1–25.

14. Office of Technology Assessment, *Payment for Physician Services: Strategies for Medicare,* OTA-H-294 (Washington, D.C.: U.S. Congress OTA, 1986).

15. M. Meiners, "Long-Term Care Insurance: Agenda for Further Research and Development," *Generations* 9 (1986):39–42.

16. W. Weissert, "Seven Reasons Why It Is so Difficult to Make Community Based Long-Term Care Cost-Effective," *Health Services Research* 20 (1985):423–433.

17. Ibid.

18. Arnett et al., "Health Spending Trends in the 1980s," 20.

19. S. Crystal, *America's Old Age Crisis: Public Policy and the Two Worlds of Aging* (New York: Basic Books, 1982).

16

The Doctor-Patient Relationship:
Traditions, Transitions, and Tensions

The current ferment in medical care involving changes in financing and organizational arrangements is a source of uncertainties and tensions. Professionals are threatened by new conditions of work that limit autonomy and earnings, but physicians as a group communicate a level of agitation that seems disproportionate to changes in their roles made necessary by newly evolving forms of organization and practice. Complaints focus on government regulation, particularly economic constraints, the legal climate particularly as it affects doctors through malpractice risk and premium increases, and growing competition from newly emerging corporate practices and a growing pool of doctors. Physician frustration is often expressed through the contention that outside parties, and government in particular, are intruding in and damaging doctor-patient relationships, and creating an adversarial context for patient care. In the stridency of debate, it is easy to discount appeals to preserving doctor-patient relationships as self-serving rhetoric. The debate may not pose the central issues most constructively, but the issue is important nevertheless.

With the enhancement of biomedical science and sophisticated technology we commonly confuse the quality of medical care with the sophistication of techniques available to the practitioner. Biomedical advances, of course, have contributed magnificently to reducing mortality among both newborns and the old and have enhanced significantly the quality of many lives. There are innumerable instances where the quality of technology may make the difference, but most commonly physicians function in situations of limited knowledge and uncertainty and depend predominantly on their clinical judgment and experience in making wise and humane decisions. Such decisions are influenced not only by the physician's competence but also by cultural attitudes and values and the incentives

236

and controls implicit in financial and organizational arrangements. The key is to understand clearly how the context either facilitates or distorts good clinical judgement, and meaningful opportunities to influence health, and the permissable tradeoffs between societal needs and values on the one hand and the specific needs and wishes of patients on the other.

The current emphasis on a competitive marketplace suggests that medical care can be equated with most other products and services. In many instances the analogy may hold. Some medical care choices, for example, are enhanced through competition such as selections among alternative health plans, purchase of drugs and appliances, and perhaps many discrete services such as simple surgical procedures. An important consideration in assessing the role of competition is the extent to which the service can be evaluated and held to a reasonably adequate standard.

The competitive model introduces tension, in particular, when the medical product is a process of sequential judgments and not a specific procedure. Such sequential judgments are the essence of much of medical care which draws not only on physicians' knowledge and clinical judgment but also on their understanding of their patients' life situations, special needs and personal tastes. Doctor-patient relationships are characterized by serious inequalities of information, and as Kenneth Arrow[1] has emphasized, the activity of medical production is the same as the product. Because the product cannot be tested before using it, and even the most informed patient cannot equal the doctor's judgment in most instances, such relationships must depend on patients' trust in the physicians' competence and that they will act in patients' best interests.

It is commonly understood that much of the value of medical care comes from the quality of association that evolves between patient and doctor, the extent the physician comes to appreciate the patients' often unstated needs and concerns, and the potential positive influence in affecting the patients' psychological well-being, improved health behavior, and adherence to an appropriate regimen. As more of medical care involves chronic disease and irreversible disability, the task of care increasingly focuses on maintaining and enhancing function and this is substantially an influence process. Good practice managing cardiac rehabilitation, treatment of cancer and stroke, or the reversal of disorientation and depression among the elderly, to choose a few examples, requires rapport and trust as well as sound knowledge and technology.

In traditional medical practice, the ethical responsibility of the doctor was to act primarily as the patient's personal agent and in the patient's interest. In reality, of course, economic and personal needs of providers and limitations of patients' resources influenced or limited treatment possibilities. But the definition of responsibility, and the expectations that is formed, set a tone for physician behavior and for the medical care process. It also provided a standard to judge departures from the norm of responsible physician behavior.

Current efforts to constrain cost typically involve modifications of two basic aspects of traditional definitions. First, they often seek to "lock-in" care to a particular physician or provider group who becomes a gatekeeper to more specialized and expensive services. Second, they change the definition of the doctor's role as primary agent of the patient to one of balancing the patient's wants and needs against a predetermined or constrainted budget. The physician or hospital role, thus, is transformed from *advocating* to *allocating*.[2] Medical care judgments are complex and not simply a response to medical training, professional ethics or economic incentives. Any plausible system we devise will respond to a mix of economic and social influences, but how we structure practice arrangements will tilt the system in different directions. In the traditional alliance, the bias was toward doing everything possible for the patient even when costs clearly exceeded benefits. New arrangements are encouraging a different calculus, and results are more difficult to anticipate.

Both types of modifications of practice arrangements potentially erode trust in subtle and even in more obvious ways. Patients feel less vulnerable when they can choose providers, sites of care and modes of treatment; and "lock-in" mechanisms make them more suspicious of the services they receive. While choice for many patients in the past has been more theoretical than real, the idea of choice strengthens the patient's confidence. The actual care may be as good in the constrained situation, but what the patient believes about care is also important. Similarly, as the physician's role is defined more in bureaucratic terms as an allocator of resources and less in terms of strong loyalty to patients, the definition of the relationship itself gives patients less reason to trust that their interests come first.

There is an irreconcilable tension between the success of cost constraint mechanisms and the extent to which doctor and patient are given discretion to work out their preferences and needs independent of competing demands. One strategy to deal with such tensions is to maintain checks and balances. In the current DRG system, for example, the fact that a strong fiscal incentive for early discharge exists for the hospital but not necessarily for the physician establishes an arena for negotiation and debate that would be less likely if they shared identical incentives. In considering extensions of DRG mechanisms for physician payment or alternative future reimbursement strategies, the value of checks and balances is worthy of attention.

Sensing the absence of any solution to the tension between individual and societal needs, some advocate that major decisions about allocation be made by external agencies, and that within these constraints, the physician's role as advocate of the patient be protected and reinforced.[3,4] The suggestion is that it is more acceptable for such decisions to be made entirely outside doctor-patient transactions. Very large and expensive changes in technological inputs should be made in a larger arena of debate and consideration, but to absolve physicians from allocative responsibility divorces decision-making from the detailed and painful contingencies of illness and disability. Our population is too large and heterogeneous, and their situations, needs and preferences too varied to allow bureaucratic officials, far from the arena of pain and anxiety, to control allocative choices. The notion that we can follow this course and retain the professional characteristics we want in physicians is in my judgment an illusion.

There is risk of exaggerating the perverse effects of new economic arrangements. Within some range of ample provision of resources, doctors will remain dedicated to patients' best interests regardless of financing arrangements, although some violations inevitably occur. All sectors of our economy are required, whether by budget limitations or the press of competitors, to establish priorities and make choices in production processes. Awareness of resource limitations and incentives to set priorities contribute to efficiency and effectiveness. The difficulty comes with increasingly severe restraints and with efforts to put individual decision-makers at sufficient personal risk that they experience their own needs in conflict with those of their patients.

Most medical care programs now in place in the United States, operating under fixed prospective budgets, such as prepaid group practices, do not put physicians at large personal risk of income loss, and this is as it should be. While these physicians probably feel constraints more than fee-for-service practitioners, and may face some administrative review and pressures, such influences are not so strong as to threaten in any fundamental way the physician's loyalty to the patient or the ability to practice medicine in an appropriate and responsible way. Moreover, the American population is sufficiently demanding, and the press sufficiently vigilant, to bring abuses to public attention. As we continue down the cost-containment path, however, efforts may be designed increasingly to put physicians at significant personal income risk. While it is constructive to put health plans and institutions at some financial risk, efforts to follow a similar course with the individual physician should be scrutinized with care.

Government should not intrude in clinical decisions but it cannot pay much of the bill and be indifferent to whether decision-making occurs within reasonable and acceptable limits. Here, there is much room for professional responsibility, and a greater willingness of physicians as a group to take renewed group and individual direction over community medical practice including protection against wastefulness, fraud and incompetence. There is a certain cynicism in the community about physician peer review and an apparent consensus that traditional peer review mechanisms have failed. Conditions have changed substantially, however, and the evaluations of peer review have focused predominantly on efficacy in cost containment. I do not believe that peer review can significantly contain aggregate costs, but it has greater potential as a mechanism to assure professional responsibility within fixed financial parameters. To the extent that peer review processes have serious administrative support, and incentives for this could be strengthened in capitation-type systems, they can play a targeted role in limiting the ability of a single physician to misuse resource pools on which other physicians depend. The role of the federal government can focus on insuring that such review processes take place and function reasonably within agreed-upon principles.

With the emphasis on cost-containment, insufficient attention has been given to improving peer review as a mechanism for physician education and as a way of increasing sensitivity to difficulties in relationships with patients and in resolving increasingly common ethical dilemmas. Moreover, providing physician groups with information on practice variations within their own contexts, and where ineffective resource allocation affects all, provides opportunities for intelligent constraints.[5] There are now increasing efforts to provide physicians feedback on their choices, and advances in computer technology and data formats make such data accessible and relatively inexpensive. Mechanisms to increase a sense of group responsibility among physicians, and making them relevant to doctor-patient conflicts that arise as new financial mechanisms come into place, require continuing developmental efforts.

There is evidence that patients are less likely to feel that doctors have interest in them when physicians work within fixed budgets, or are paid by salary or capitation and not directly by the patient.[6] Most patients, in most contexts, remain satisfied, and the difference is only one of degree. As the need to control expenditures increases the tensions between patient and physician interests, however, we will need sophisticated ways to settle disputes without resorting to litigation. A strong peer review system, viewed by the community as legitimate, could contribute toward resolving many difficulties in less formal ways than either formal grievance mechanisms or the litigation process.

Government must set financial constraints but should not micro-manage the care system. No social policy can be sufficiently sophisticated to anticipate and make provision for the inevitable clinical cases that depart from the norm. Moreover, centralized authority, however benevolent, is isolated from the pain, worry, uncertainty, and disruption that characterize serious illness. It too easily loses touch with the feelings of patients and their families and the tone of interaction. Government can contribute, however, to a framework of trust by providing for patient choice among alternative health care systems and types of care, by facilitating the ability of public recipients to change their source of care if dissatisfied, and providing accessible and simple modes of resolution for grievances. Each of these mechanisms communicates to participants some sense of control and contributes to their confidence in the system.

Tensions in the medical care process are an inevitable consequence of the successes of biomedical knowledge and technology relative to our economic incapacities to do all we know. We accept such tensions in all other aspects of our lives and we will learn to accept them in medicine as well. These tensions cannot be eliminated, and depending on how they are structured, can contribute to thoughtful choices. My view is that such tensions must be resolved at the individual level, between doctor and patient, and client and health care plan. A framework must evolve that allows doctor and patient sufficient latitude to work out different needs and tastes consistent with the heterogeneity of our population. These differences can be resolved best if negotiations take place within a framework of choice. The patient's and doctor's awareness of options remains the most simple means to minimize tension and promote constructive dialogue.

References

1. Arrow K. J. Uncertainty and the welfare economics of medical care. Am Econ Rev. 1963; 53:941–73.
2. Mechanic D. From advocacy to allocation: The evolving American health care system. New York: The Free Press, 1986.
3. Fried C. Rights and health care—Beyond equity and efficiency. N Engl J Med. 1975; 293: 241–45.
4. Daniels N. Why saying no to patients in the United States is so hard. N Engl J Med. 1986; 314: 1380–83.
5. Wennberg J. E. Dealing with medical practice variations: A proposal for action. Heal Aff. 1984; 3:6–32.
6. Luft H. Health maintenance organizations: Dimensions of performance. New York: Wiley-Interscience, 1981.

17

Future Challenges in Health and Health Care

In that classic tale delighting adults and children alike, Alice asks, "Would you tell me, please, which way I ought to go from here?" "That depends a good deal on where you want to get to," said the cat.

In examining specific issues and solutions it is probably useful to step back and reconsider more simply what we seek from medical care. A major characteristic of the gigantic health industry—with its vast array of health workers, facilities, technologies, entitlement and insurance programs, reimbursement mechanisms and competing alternatives—is the tendency for individual components to assume a life of their own, made possible by decentralized planning and the opportunities available through a complex reimbursement process. In focusing on specific issues and debates, it is relatively easy to lose sight of overall objectives.

The future of health care in the United States will undoubtedly evolve by building on existing forms of organization, traditional professional groupings, and dominant types of facilities. Only by having a strong sense of purpose and direction can we shape significantly what now exists in more constructive directions. Many biomedical developments are to be applauded, but the distortions in the total pattern of health care services, and the limited accomplishments for some very large investments are striking. There is no assurance that careful priorities will prevail over economic, political and technological imperatives in any instance, but it is apparent that if we lack a clear conception of our goals, there is not much chance of competing successfully with the powerful, persistent, and motivated interests that frequent the health care arena. Health care is big business, and those who wish to shape it as a start need a clear vision, well thought out strategies and a great deal of persistence.

How then, do we define the mission of this large, powerful and expanding industry? Health is, of course, ultimately its object. The World Health

Organization's (WHO) definition of health as a state of "complete physical, mental and social well-being," however, strikes the pragmatist as utopian and divorced from the hard realities. But it alerts us to two important conclusions. First, health is shaped fundamentally by culture, society and environment and it is mostly at the margins that medical care services have their primary impact. Most of the great advances in health status arise from basic improvements in economic status, education, nutrition, lifestyles and the environment. Medical care is an important influence, but only one of many. Second, the WHO statement attunes us to the fact that physical illness and psychological discomfort, however influenced by inheritance and biology, arise in no small way from conditions in the family, at work, and in the community more generally. Patients' experiences of illness reflect both responses to noxious influences and ways of adapting to intolerable stresses that tax their capabilities and spirit. The biology and psychology of health are inextricably interconnected.

Medical care, of course, is a more narrow concern than health enhancement, but its goals must be broad. Health care professionals have responsibility to support and sustain those suffering pain, distress and incapacity and to restore patients to their maximal potential of functioning. The words may sound trite and unnecessary, but the fact is that most medical care is more directed to diagnosis and management of specific disease than to considering how to restore functioning or to assist patients most appropriately within the context of their illnesses and disabilities if cure is elusive. While remarkable progress has been made in the past by pursuing limited concepts of cause and a narrow view of the physician's responsibilities, the changing age profile of the population and emerging patterns of illness and disability suggest that the challenge for future health professionals will be less with cure and more with maintaining function. It gives us pause to reflect on the fact that the fastest growing subgroup of senior citizens are those over 85. This subgroup increased 174 percent between 1960 and 1980 and is expected to increase another 110 percent between 1980 and the year 2000.

These increases among the old-old in part reflect the fact that the American population is healthier than ever before, and even the majority of the now more numerous elderly maintain their function and vitality. On a statistical basis, most serious disease does not occur with frequency until relatively late in life, is chronic rather than acute, and poses serious issues for life routines, work and adaptation for those affected. Elderly patients with chronic problems constitute an increasing proportion of the typical physician's workload and occupancy on inpatient medical or surgical services. For many the issue is not cure, but how to live in a satisfactory fashion with chronic disease and the impediments it presents.

A Necessary Balance

Medical care thus must balance carefully two competing opportunities. Thinking epidemiologically, the burden of illness falls on the elderly and the impaired, and the major challenge is to ameliorate suffering and promote functioning. But the increasing sophistication of the sciences relevant to medicine and the perfection of new technologies and procedures also makes it possible to serve the population in new and dramatic ways. When thought of in terms of knowledge development, new biomedical technology offers possibilities of serving patients in more effective ways. But when new and unproven technologies, or those whose costs outweigh their benefits, are carried forward as an imperative they raise frightening issues of financing, questions about the actual welfare achieved, and tough conflicts about the payoffs in pursuing elusive cures at the neglect of care.

In sharp contrast to impressive technical advances are continuing complaints among the chronically ill that health professionals are inattentive and often show a lack of interest in issues of functioning and the quality of their lives, which is of greatest concern to them.

The young middle-aged man following a myocardial infarction and his spouse are vitally interested in his capacity to return to work, support, his family, and maintain a normal marital relationship. Relevant questions are typically evaded or ignored, or the instruction provided is so vague as to be unhelpful and increases rather than reduces anxiety and anger. Too often the medical focus is on small changes in cardiac output and far too little attention is given to the patient's social well-being. These are not costly efforts in technology or in the medical care process. But they take time, interest and patience and the acquisition of the necessary knowledge and sensitivity to be truly helpful.

A couple of years ago Dr. DeWitt Stetten, Jr., a distinguished physician and science administrator, wrote about his own frustrating experiences in coping with his increasing blindness resulting from macular degeneration. Although himself a physician, dedicated throughout his career to the enhancement of biomedical science, he discovered how little he was assisted by physicians who were interested in vision but not in blindness. Stetten writes: "Through all these years, and despite many contacts with skilled and experienced professionals, no ophthalmologist has at any time suggested any devices that might be of assistance to me. No ophthalmologist has mentioned any of the many ways in which I could stem the deterioration in the quality of my life.''

While the observation can be replicated in every waiting room and hospital service, what makes this observation particularly remarkable and . poignant is that it comes from a physician who dedicated his professional life to the enhancement of the best science base possible in medical practice. But the sciences relevant to the practice of medicine include sociology and psychology and their applications as much as molecular biology and immunology.

No sensible person denigrates the remarkable contributions of science to enhancing medical care, or those yet to come in the future. But good science, prudently applied, must relate to a larger framework of goals, priorities and ethics. It is the mindless uses of science, and not science itself, that deflect our basic goals.

Among values about medical care, access for all stands particularly high and symbolically represents our nation's commitment to assist the fulfillment of the individual's personal and social choices and our social commitment to equal opportunity. We share ·the value that provision of necessary services should reflect need and not the ability to pay. Following this view, governmental has made efforts to facilitate access for the old, the poor, and the medically indigent, and has struggled to develop a framework for equitable allocation that was remarkably successful in the 1960s and 1970s as measured by improvements in physician and, hospital access, and measures of disability, disease specific mortality, and longevity. We must guard against losing the ground so painstakingly acquired in the past couple of decades.

Painful Choices

Current pressures to contain costs, and how we deal with them, confront us with issues of priorities and values and perhaps painful choices as well. During times of financial stress the groups easiest to disenfranchise and the programs easiest to cut are those involving the poor and disabled. Largely dependent on public funds, with poorly organized constituencies to protect existing entitlements, they are vulnerable to federal, state and local government limits on eligibility, cutbacks in the range of available services, and imposition of significant and often prohibitive cost sharing requirements. The same decision-makers that impose these burdens will permit and even encourage the application of expensive technical innovations of limited benefit that in some cases, as for example, hemodialysis among the very old, are often used inappropriately. It is ironic that the unproven uses of technology expand at the same time that we limit basic care for the poor and the chronically handicapped as well as opportunities for prevention, patient education and rehabilitation assistance.

Dependency requires that we maintain access to a reasonable level of health care services for all, and there is a strong and persistent national consensus that government should insure that result. There is also a commonly shared perception in the population—evident in almost every patient care survey—that patients desire professionals who direct attention to their broad needs, who demonstrate a personal interest in them and treat them without a sense of haste, who allow them to ask questions and provide responsive and informative feedback, and who treat illness in a way that facilitates and promotes fulfillment of usual activities.

Hospitalized patients in particular have a variety of needs related to their illnesses and to their overall well-being that may be as important to the ultimate outcome as specific medical interventions. Important from a social perspective is determining the least restrictive treatment regimen and teaching patients to manage their lives to minimize illness-related disabilities and to cope with various contingencies and uncertainties. Patients need opportunities to experiment with aspects of the treatment regimen, and to obtain informative and supportive feedback. When a variety of medical and other health personnel are involved in the patient's hospital care, there is a further need for effective and consistent communication with the patient and with staff to minimize contradictions, duplication of efforts, unnecessary anxieties, and confusions and breakdowns in the processes of care.

In the context of economic pressures, the preservation of access or the types of responsiveness I have described cannot be taken for granted, nor are existing incentives consistent with emphasis on the socio-emotional, interpersonal, or educational components of care that play a major role in maintaining function. Present reimbursement, in contrast, encourages technical discrete procedures and induces competition and conflict among varying providers and professionals.

The transition, however slow, toward capitated payment and fixed reimbursement impresses me as the only assured way to cope with cost dilemmas in a way that allows more careful balancing among care options, types of professional services, and treatment settings. The future potential of physician assistants, nurse practitioners, and other non-physician health professionals who devote a great deal of time and effort to caring functions is much more likely to be realized in financial contexts where decisions about types of services, personnel and technologies must be weighed relative to both treatment goals and total resources available for care.

In capitated contexts, the fact that such professionals provide services comparable to those of the physician at less cost and often with greater patient satisfaction would strongly argue for their increased use. With the impending growth of the physician supply, the future of these health professionals and many of the unique services they provide are in jeopardy without a more neutral reimbursement structure that requires that the role and value of their services be weighted against other expenditures. There is every indication that Americans will support generous expenditures for medical care, but distortions of dominant payment mechanisms make it likely that the poorest and most needy patients will be most disadvantaged and that the less powerful professional groups whose work overlaps with tasks carried out by physicians will be held in check, if not increasingly disenfranchised.

Neutral Incentive System

Since most of health care is uncertain, establishing goals by regulation is a dangerous, if not a hopeless, task. We can, however, more readily develop an incentive system of greater neutrality, one that encourages careful assessments of tradeoffs among sites of care, appropriate professional providers, mix of services and intensity of care. Government constraints cannot intelligently provide guidance except in the most general ways, but they can provide the incentives that would insure that such evaluations take place. The only mechanism that achieves this without extensive and intrusive regulation is an established budget.

An established budget is initially more neutral than any other form of payment because it leaves priority judgments to administrative and professional decision-making. While the size of the budget involves the value judgment of how much is medical care worth, this is appropriately a political decision that should be made in a context of considering other major needs and sectors as well. Politics do not necessarily result in the wisest decisions, but they provide the proper forum for the necessary public discussion.

Health professionals, in contrast, are best prepared to assess, given a budget, how it might reasonably be allocated to achieve desired objectives for a defined population. There is no assurance that they will do it well or in a manner divorced from their particular interests, biases and preferences. But their judgments, however colored by their special perspectives, are still preferable to those established in some uniform way by bureaucratic officials far from the scene of action and who can abstractly divorce themselves from the pain, worry and uncertainty associated with serious illness and incapacity.

The inappropriateness of current payment mechanisms is due not only to their distorting qualities, but even more to their specific biases in favoring hospital care to outpatient services, technical to cognitive approaches and heroic curative efforts to efforts to promote functioning and morale. Fixed budgets are no panacea, and will not do away with ingrained preferences to solve the esoteric, overcome the difficult challenge, or to be intrigued by the more interesting or attractive patient. But the constraint of such a budget demands managerial and professional consideration of a more cost-effective mix between physicians and other professionals, and a better opportunity to balance some medical social services and other essential human services against costly and sometimes inappropriate technical ones.

The goals and prescriptions I have described are difficult, but neither radical nor impossible. The pressures to protect the economic position of the rapidly increasing corps of physicians will encourage the most blatant protectionism and reactionary stances to innovations in organizing services and in the use of non-medical practitioners. Physicians, resisting the intrusions on their autonomy by large corporations and hospitals on the one hand, the increasingly powerful competing health professional groups seeking to maintain and enhance their positions on the other, may not be models of reason in the unfolding public debate.

The fact, however we disguise it, is that American health care is now predominantly a publicly financed activity with major economic, social and political ramifications for all of us. It increasingly competes with much else we value in the context of a zero-sum society. The public that pays the bills would be foolish to allow those who collect the purse to establish the objects of the enterprise or the framework of the impending debate. To borrow a phrase from the late René Dubos, I would describe myself as a despairing optimist on these issues. The powerful interests are clearly evident and I'm not foolish enough to see a resolution coming easily. But I know that if the many talented and dedicated health professionals and other important actors in this arena make the effort to achieve an equitable and responsive solution, American health care can be the envy of the entire world.